Intermittent Fa
Women Over 50

The guide to lose weight without hunger pangs and increase your energy, 8 techniques that led me to success + 101 mouth-watering recipes and a 14-day eating plan.

Jean Eenfeldt

Dear Reader,

i am a 56 year old woman, born and raised in America and currently living in Lakewood. I lost a total of 140 pounds (65 kilos) from my highest weight. It took me two years to lose the weight, and I have since maintained the loss for over a year and a half.

I started my weight loss journey with calorie restriction, while continuing to eat carbs. I lost some weight, but soon stalled for many months. The lack of progress almost broke me, and I felt like giving up. After much research online, I discovered the intermittent diet. I made sure to learn the science behind the intermittent diet by watching many YouTube videos, reading books on the intermittent diet, and using websites for personal research

I decided to trust the process and the science before giving up completely.... And so, I tried the intermittent.

In the past, I had tried every diet known to man and failed.

So, when I started reading about intermittent dieting, it seemed crazy. After decades of rejecting fat and believing that you can't live without carbs, I couldn't understand the aspect on time windows and decided to trust the process and the science before giving up completely....

So, I tried the intermittent diet.

As soon as I started in February 2019, the weight started dropping once again (slowly but surely), and I started feeling much better and healthier. I no longer had carb-crashing afternoon naps.

I felt energized throughout the day, had great focus, my skin cleared up, and I lost weight and inches. Most importantly, my high blood pressure, which I had suffered from for decades, was finally reversed within a few months and has normalized to this day without medication.

I was also amazed that within the first month of complete intermittent eating, even the painful menstrual cramps I had suffered from for decades completely disappeared. There are still so many more benefits you'll find within my book and long story short, the intermittent diet has completely changed my life.

For the first time in my life, I feel good about myself physically, emotionally, and mentally. I have the energy of a young girl again.

On top of that, it is the easiest and tastiest "diet" I have ever done in my life. In fact, the only hard part was the patience part - as would be the case with any weight loss journey because it's a marathon, not a race - but I took the journey one day at a time, telling myself just for today, I'll eat well, and a few days turned into a week, then a month, and now years. These days, I look back and feel so grateful for taking the chance and sticking with it...there were some stalling moments, but I kept telling myself to keep going no matter what, and during those stalling moments, I still saw the loss of inches and felt the clothes looser.

I've lost most of my weight from my upper body, which makes me realize that a lot of the visceral fat surrounding my vital organs has melted away. I have a waist for the first time in my life and now wear a belt with my clothes and enjoy shopping for fashionable clothes (and not just anything that fits like I used to).

Since February 2019, I've been eating this way, and now I know I can eat sustainably for the rest of my life. I love having the fatty cuts of meat along with the non-starchy vegetables. Being able to salt, cook in delicious butter and coconut oil, and pour olive oil on my salads is amazing. I always feel full and full for hours after a meal. I never feel deprived.

When I did that initial research, I realized the science of insulin resistance was solid. Especially for people who have struggled with weight issues for decades, perhaps since early childhood, and couldn't lose weight with low-calorie diets, as in my case.

Once I started the intermittent diet, the food cravings I'd always had completely disappeared, and I've been cured of my addiction to binge eating for years now.

This way of eating works. It is the key to breaking a lifetime's struggles with food addiction and can reverse lifestyle diseases.

I can say that with the loss of 140 pounds (64 kilos), my life has completely transformed for the better and I have regained my health by leaps and bounds. I am also active now and go to the gym four to five times a week for strength training and cardio. However, throughout the journey, I have been 90-95% focused on food and have only used exercise as an adjunct for heart health. This way of eating works if you trust the process.

I am thankful for this diet and like many others who are spreading awareness of the benefits of this lifestyle I chose to tell you my story to help you and get back to living your LIFE.

Knowledge is power, and I hope the world can open their eyes and see the health benefits of this lifestyle.

Kind regards,

Jean

Table of Contents

How Does It Work 19

The Science Behind Intermittent Fasting 22

The Practice of Fasting Through the Course of Human History 23

Differences in Metabolism Between a Young Woman and a Healthy Over 50 27

Intermittent Fasting and Longevity 30

Intermittent Fasting Boosts Productivity 31

Fasting Is Dangerous 32

Fasting Can Lower Your Blood Sugar Dangerously 32

It Will Cause Hormonal Imbalance 33

It Will Destroy Your Metabolism 33

It Causes Stress 34

Fasting Can Lead to Overeating 34

Fasting Causes the Body to Burn Muscle 35

You Can't Work Out While Fasting 35

Getting Started Takes an Adjustment 36

Potential to Overeat..37

Possible Leptin Imbalance 37

You May Become Dehydrated..37

Not Everyone Can Practice Intermittent Fasting...................38

It Can Trigger the Re-Feeding Syndrome 39

Having Low Energy 39

Interfere With the Social Side of Eating 39

Reproductive Complications in Some Women 40

Digestive Complications..40

Weight Regains...41

16/8 Method..42

Lean-Gains Method (14:10)..43

20:4 Method..44

Meal Skipping 45

Warrior Diet Fasting..46

Eat-Stop-Eat (24 Hour) Method 47

Alternate-Day Method...48

12:12 Method..49

The Mindset for Success...50

9

Set Goals 53

Plan Your Portions 55

A Step-by-Step Approach 56

The Best Tips and Tricks for Starting Intermittent Fasting.... 59

Intermittent Fasting and Exercise 61

Mistakes to Avoid During Intermittent Fasting Diet 69

Foods to Embrace 81

Foods to Avoid 83

Nutrition Plan 86

Stick to the Same Foods 87

Carbs 87

Post Meal Hunger 87

How to Combine the Two 89

Benefits of the Keto Diet When You're Fasting 90

Breakfast Recipes 92

Lunch Recipes 97

Dinner Recipes 102

Appetizers and Snacks 107

Salads and Soups 112

Meat Recipes 116

Fish Recipes 123

Superfoods for Women Over 50 129

Week 1 134

Week 2 136

Is Intermittent Fasting Difficult to Adhere To? 138

What Is the Recommended Number of Hours/Days for Fasting? 138

Do I Still Need to Count Calories? 138

Should Women Do IF Differently?.................................... 139

Is It Safe for Pregnant or Breastfeeding Women to Fast?.. 139

Can I Still Work Out Even If I Am Doing IF?...................... 140

© **Copyright 2021 - Jean Eenfeldt -All rights reserved**.

This document is geared towards providing exact and reliable information in regard to the topic and issue covered.

- From a Declaration of Principles which was accepted and approved equally by a Committee of the American Bar Association and a Committee of Publishers and Associations.

In no way is it legal to reproduce, duplicate, or transmit any part of this document in either electronic means or in printed format. All rights reserved.

The information provided herein is stated to be truthful and consistent, in that any liability, in terms of inattention or otherwise, by any usage or abuse of any policies, processes, or directions contained within is the solitary and utter responsibility of the recipient reader. Under no circumstances will any legal responsibility or blame be held against the publisher for any reparation, damages, or monetary loss due to the information herein, either directly or indirectly.

Respective authors own all copyrights not held by the publisher.

The information herein is offered for informational purposes solely and is universal as so. The presentation of the information is without contract or any type of guarantee assurance.
The trademarks that are used are without any consent, and the publication of the trademark is without permission or backing by the trademark owner. All trademarks and brands within this book are for clarifying purposes only and are owned by the owners themselves, not affiliated with this document.

Introduction

Our way of life and eating habits undoubtedly affect our health. Too much sugar, alcohol, stress, medications, and poor eating habits create a firm foundation for developing disease and illness. More so, it causes us to be necessarily obese, gaining excessive weight and causing a kind of limitation to our lifestyle. However, with fasting, we get the chance to activate our internal healing force, which helps to detoxify, cleanse, and rebalance the body, prevent and cure diseases, and renew energy.

In principle, intermittent fasting is not new in terms of religions and customs. Intermittent fasting has also been on everyone's lips for some time.

Lack of exercise and the constant availability of healthy dieting has had an extremely unfavorable impact on our health over the past few decades: affluent diseases, like overweight, cardiovascular diseases, and type 2 diabetes are increasing dramatically.

A little exercise and the excessive consumption of sugar and carbohydrates are entirely unnatural for evolution: The "primeval man" as a hunter and gatherer always had periods of fasting because the food was not always available. The interval fasting system is based on this original type of nutrition.

In contrast to conventional fasting or therapeutic fasting, intermittent fasting is not entirely dispensed with but only fasted part-time. The phases of healthy eating and complete waiving alternate, depending on the method, for short or long intervals. A regular diet is quite crucial for intermittent fasting. If the food is missing for too long, the body switches to hunger metabolism, which results in a slowdown in metabolism and a decrease in general calorie consumption. The result is reduced weight loss and muscle breakdown.

Based on all this information, nutritional experts around the world agree that IF (as Intermittent Fasting would be referred to in most of this book) is less stressful for our bodies than many other diets.

When a woman approaches a certain age, her body starts changing as the aging process kicks in. Women over 50 become high-risk targets for various health issues and start to find it harder to maintain their weight.

There has been scientific interest in intermittent fasting as research has started to uncover its numerous benefits. Post-menopause causes many changes in a woman, including increased belly fat, depression, muscle pain, and joint pain.

Women are moreover at more considerable risk for diabetes and cardiovascular disease.

Research has shown that intermittent fasting in women over 50 could possibly reduce the risk of diabetes and may ease muscle and joint pain, especially lower back pain. It could, in addition, produce a positive anti-aging effect which is a bonus along with better weight control to cut down on belly fat.

Trust me; you wouldn't want to be left out of it to ensure that you "stop dieting and start living" to ensure that you maintain a good weight and body balance... Let's go!

Chapter 1. What Is Intermittent Fasting?

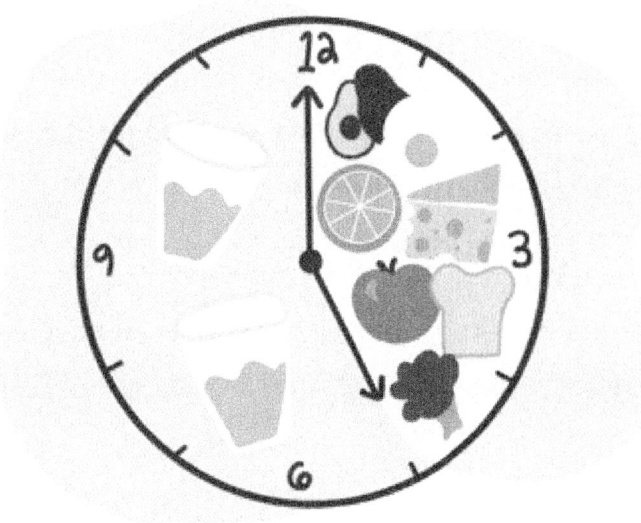

Basically, fasting is defined as abstaining from eating anything. It is the deliberate action of depriving the body of any form of food for more than six hours.

Whereas Intermittent fasting is a nutritional strategy that provides for a more or less long interval of fasting over a few days, alternating with a period in which you can take food without being too enslaved to the weights but still taking into account some precautions. Intermittent fasting does not need to be carried out every day, but you can choose the different ways suitable for your goals and lifestyles.

In the hours of feeding it is possible to consume almost all foods giving preference to low-calorie foods such as meat, fish, eggs, limiting simple sugars and choosing those with a low glycemic index, bread, pasta, and rice possibly whole grains, legumes, dried and fresh fruits, good fats.

One of its forms is where the fast is carried out in a cyclic manner with the aim to reduce the overall caloric intake in a day.

The main goal is to divert the body's attention from the digestion of food. During the fasting period, in fact, a series of metabolic changes take place in the body: since there is no food left in the stomach to digest, the body focuses on the process of recovery and maintenance.

To most people, it may sound unhealthy and damaging for the body, but scientific research has proven that fasting can produce positive results on the human mind and body. According to Healthline, the American medical-scientific journal, this system helps reduce overall calorie intake and as a result not only can help people lose weight effortlessly but can improve the overall functioning of metabolism. It can also positively affect our mind teaching self-discipline and fighting against bad eating practices and habits. It is basically an umbrella term that is used to define all voluntary forms of fasting. This dietary approach does not restrict the consumption of certain food items; rather, it works by reducing the overall food intake, leaving enough space to meet the essential nutrients the body needs. Therefore, it is proven to be far more effective and much easier in implementation, given that the dieter completely understands the nature and science of intermittent fasting.

Intermittent fasting is categorized into three broad methods of food abstinence, including alternate-day fasting, daily restrictions, and periodic fasting. The means may vary, but the end goal of intermittent fasting remains the same, which is to achieve a better metabolism, healthy body weight, and active lifestyle. The American Heart Association, AHA, has also studied intermittent fasting and its results. According to the AHA, it can help in countering insulin resistance, cardio-metabolic diseases, and leads to weight loss. However, a question mark remains on the sustainability of this health-effective method. The 2019 research "Effects of intermittent fasting on health, aging, and disease" has also found intermittent fasting to be effective against insulin resistance, inflammation, hypertension, obesity, and dyslipidemia. However, the work on this dietary approach is still underway, and the traditional methods of fasting which existed for almost the entire human history, in every religion from Buddhism to Jainism, Orthodox Christianity, Hinduism, and Islam, are studied to found relevance in today's age of science and technology.

How Does It Work

Eating is a primary need that we satisfy unceasingly from birth. Every day we introduce food into our organisms. When we eat, the metabolism activates itself to start the digestive process.

When we fast, however, we stop this process and this energy dispensing. The saved energy is thus diverted to other metabolic processes, essentially of a restorative type.

Dr. Longo, Director of the Institute of Longevity at the University of Southern California, explained how, thanks to this practice: "the immune system frees itself from useless, unnecessary cells, while it is driven to put back into action naturally, as was the case at the moments of birth and growth, stem cells capable of ensuring regeneration".

The body not engaged in food digestion can better devote itself to its purification by moving toxins away through its emunctory organs. These large internal cleanings obviously have positive repercussions on the state of health of organs and tissues. The organism is detoxified and revitalized.

American researchers at Yale's School of Medicine highlighted how during the break from food, our organism produces a substance capable of extinguishing chronic inflammation. It is called the β-hydroxybutyrate (BHB) and it is capable turn falls into a complex set of proteins that guide the inflammatory response in many pathologies, including several autoimmune diseases. A good result suggests how in the future therapeutic fasting can be used in the early treatment of many inflammatory-based diseases.

In fact, it works between alternating periods of eating and fasting. It is a much more flexible approach, as there are many options to choose from according to body type, size, weight goals, and nutritional needs.

The human body works like a synchronized machine that requires sufficient time for self-healing and repair. When we constantly eat junk and unhealthy food or too high a quantity of food without the consideration of our caloric needs, it leads to obesity and toxic build-up in the body. That is why fasting comes as a natural means of detoxifying the body and providing it enough time to utilize its fat deposits.

Whatever the human body consumes is ultimately broken into glucose, which is later utilized by the cells in glycolysis to release energy. Intermittent fasting seems to reverse this process by deliberately creating energy deprivation, which is then fulfilled by breaking down the existing fat deposits.

Intermittent fasting works through lipolysis; though it is a natural body process, it can only be initiated when the blood glucose levels drop to a sufficiently low point. That point can be achieved through fasting and exercising. When a person cuts off the external glucose supply for several hours, the body switches to lipolysis. This process of breaking the fats also releases other by-products like ketones which are capable of reducing the oxidative stress of the body and help in its detoxification.

Mark Mattson, a neuroscientist from Johns Hopkins Medicine University, has studied intermittent fasting for almost 25 years of his career. He laid out the workings of intermittent fasting by clarifying its clinical application and the science behind it. According to him, intermittent fasting must be pursued for a healthy lifestyle.

While discussing the application of this dietary approach, it is imperative to understand how intermittent fasting stands out from casual dieting practices. It is not mere abstinence from eating. What is eaten in this dietary lifestyle is equally important as the fasting itself. It does not result in malnutrition; rather, it promotes healthy eating along with the fast. Intermittent fasting is divided into two different states that follow one another. The cycle starts with the "FED" state, which is followed by a "Fasting" state. The duration of the fasting state and the frequency of the FED state are established by the method of intermittent fasting. The latter is characterized by high blood glucose levels, whereas during the fasting state the body goes through a gradual decline in glucose levels. This decline in glucose signals the pancreas and the brain to meet the body's energy needs by processing the available fat molecules. However, if the fasting state is followed by a FED state in which a person binge eats food rich in carbs and fats, it will turn out to be more hazardous for their health. Therefore, the fasting period must be accompanied by a healthy diet.

The Science Behind Intermittent Fasting

Biologically, intermittent fasting works at many levels, from cellular levels to gene expression and body growth. In order to understand the science behind the workings of intermittent fasting, it is important to learn about the role of insulin levels, human growth hormones, cellular repair, and gene expression. Intermittent fasting firstly lowers glucose levels, which in turn drops insulin levels. This lowering of insulin helps fat burning in the body, thus gradually curbing obesity and related disorders. Controlled levels of insulin are also responsible for preventing diabetes and insulin resistance. On the other hand, intermittent fasting boosts the production of human growth hormones up to five times. The increased production of HGH aids quick fat burning and muscle formation.

During the fasting state, the body goes into the process of self-healing at cellular levels, thus removing the unwanted, unfunctional cells and debris. This creates a cleansing effect that directly or indirectly nourishes the body and allows it to grow under reduced oxidative stress. Likewise, fasting even affects the gene expression within the human body. The cell functions according to the coding and decoding of the gene's expression; when this transcription occurs at a normal pace in a healthy environment, it automatically translates into the longevity of the cells, and fasting ensures unhindered transcription. Thus, intermittent fasting fights aging, cancer, and boosts the immune system by strengthening the body cells.

The Practice of Fasting Through the Course of Human History

Fasting is an ancient tradition and time-tested approach. It is one of the best tools to lose weight. It also improves concentration, prevents Alzheimer's, extends life, controls insulin resistance levels, and reverses the aging process. It is not a new concept. People have just forgotten it. Everything we eat increases the level of insulin to a certain extent. Eating healthy foods prevents those high levels. Some food items are much better than others, but they all still increase the level of insulin. The only key to avert resistance levels is to sustain low insulin levels. If they all raise insulin levels, then voluntary abstinence is the best answer, i.e. fasting.

The practice of fasting has therapeutically been used since the 5th century BC, when Hippocrates, a Greek physician, suggested abstinence from drink or food for his patients who had certain symptoms of an illness. Some called it fasting, others believed that patients naturally lost appetite in certain diseases. Some people thought that managing eating levels during such conditions were unnecessary. But many people believed that fasting was an essential and natural way to recover. An in-depth understanding of fasting and its physiological effects moved towards the evolutionary road later in the 19th century—studies organized for the first time on humans and animals.

In the early 20th century, much was known and studied about nutrition. The nutritional needs and requirements of a human body were studied in detail, and some different, new approaches to fasting emerged.

There were also some other approaches, modified fasting, which allowed an intake of 200–500 calories a day and included spiritual or psychological therapy. Depending on the form of fasting method that was being used, calories were in the shape of bread, fruit juice, honey, milk, or vegetable broth. The modified fasting approach was different from a diet having low calories that allowed a maximum of 800 calories a day. It had the primary purpose of losing weight. On the other hand, intermittent fasting involved calorie restriction in cyclic periods like 12 hours of fasting plan followed by 12 hours of regular consumption of calories.

The ancient people, especially Greeks, considered nature as a guiding force in their medical treatment. According to them, fasting was undoubtedly one of the best traditions of ancient healing in human history, and it improved the cognitive abilities of a person. Many religions and cultures have practiced it. But, keep in mind that fasting is very much different from starvation. Fasting is about voluntarily holding back from food. Starvation, on the other hand, is an involuntary action. You probably have no control over it. People with starvation do not have the choice of deciding the time of their next meal. They do not even know if that time will ever come or not. So, do not confuse these terms.

Fasting was also supported by many intellectual giants like Philip Paracelsus, who is the father of toxicology. He considered fasting an excellent remedy, and called it the "physician within". Benjamin Franklin, who had a wide range of knowledge and intellect in various areas, also called fasting the best medicine, along with resting. Fasting has also served the spiritual purpose of many religions. Religious leaders like Buddha, Jesus Christ, and prophet Muhammed shared one common belief of considering fasting as a healing power. It is also called purification or cleansing in a spiritual context. But fasting developed differently and independently among these cultures and religions as something profound and intrinsically beneficial.

In Buddhism, people consume food just in the morning time and do fasting from noon to the next day morning. On the other hand, Muslims choose the time from the sunrise to the sunset in their holy month, Ramadan. Prophet Muhammad used to encourage fasting on other days of the week, too, except Ramadan. The fasting in Ramadan is different from other fasting protocols. The use of fluids is also forbidden during this fast. So, they include a little bit of mild dehydration in their fast too.

So, the idea of fasting has genuinely evolved. Many influential people have agreed that fasting is a truly beneficial approach for a healthy life. As discussed, fasting has a long history, but various aspects of why and how we should do have changed drastically. Modern approaches towards intermittent fasting comprise of fasting periods regularly occurring in between the eating periods. You can eat healthy food. The approach is to do it by sticking to a small-time frame, the eating window, and staying away from food in the fasting window. Today, we have absolute freedom to select any form of fasting. The intermittent fast lasts from 6–24 hours of an extended period. You can go for a fast for just one day in a week, a month, or a year. You can select the shorter fast approach or, the longer one. You will not find one specific best approach to fasting. It is a very personal preference and experience. It is just simple, effective, and practical.

Chapter 2.   The Best Diet for Women Over 50

Differences in Metabolism Between a Young Woman and a Healthy Over 50

At the most basic level, it must be said that there are detailed bodily differences between young women and older women. Many of these bodily differences become obvious with the outward, physical effects of aging, but a lot of them also happen on the inside, away from what our eyes can see.

When women age, enter and exit menopause, and become fully mature, their bodies change, reflecting different nutritional needs for the next 30+ years. During menopause, in particular, certain foods help with the urges, hot flashes, and more, but the period of intense transition is more of a gateway into a completely altered future (mentally, bodily, nutritionally, and more).

Women of this age experience slowed metabolism (to their great frustrations) as well as lowered hormone production. For weight and mood, therefore, menopause and maturation are equal disasters. Your body will go completely "out of whack," compared to how it used to function. You'll likely put on weight despite the dietary choices you make, and you may feel there's no relief in sight. Don't be fooled, however! Things may have changed for you, but they won't be stagnant changes.

Essentially, women at the stage of menopause and beyond need to absorb less energy overall from their food, yet they need more protein to deal with the effects of aging. Vitamins B12 and D, calcium, and zinc will need to be boosted, while iron becomes less important for the aging female body. Vitamins C, E, A, and beta-carotene need to be increased too in order to fight off cancer, infection, disease, and more.

As the woman ages and matures even further, more things will change; mainly, she cannot bypass taking these important supplements any longer. In older and more mature women, the body's abilities to recognize hunger and thirst become muted, and dehydration poses a greater threat. Fewer calories are required for the older and more mature woman too, but she still needs to get as many nutrients as (if not more than!) the young woman does.

It seems that a younger woman can eat (relatively) what she wants and not worry about taking vitamins or supplements, but it is undeniable that the older woman will need this nutritional help to ensure longevity. Basically, health needs become more pressing for women at this age, as their bodies are less flexible and resistant to problems that may arise.

How IF Affects Women at This Age and How to Approach It

Because health, diet, reproductivity, and nutritional needs are all altered for mature and menopausal women, their relationships with intermittent fasting can be very different from young women. For instance, while young women ought to be careful about how intermittent fasting can affect their fertility levels, older women can practice intermittent fasting freely without these concerns. Therefore, more mature women can apply the weight-loss techniques of intermittent fasting to their lives (and waistlines) without the worry of what negative side-effects might arise in the future.

For menopausal women, however, the situation is a little bit different than it is for fully mature women. People going through menopause have to deal with daily hormone fluctuations that cause hot and cold flashes, sleeplessness, anxiety, irregular periods, and more. At the beginning of this process, intermittent fasting will not necessarily help, and it could even make your situation more stressful.

Chapter 3. Benefits of IF for Women Over 50

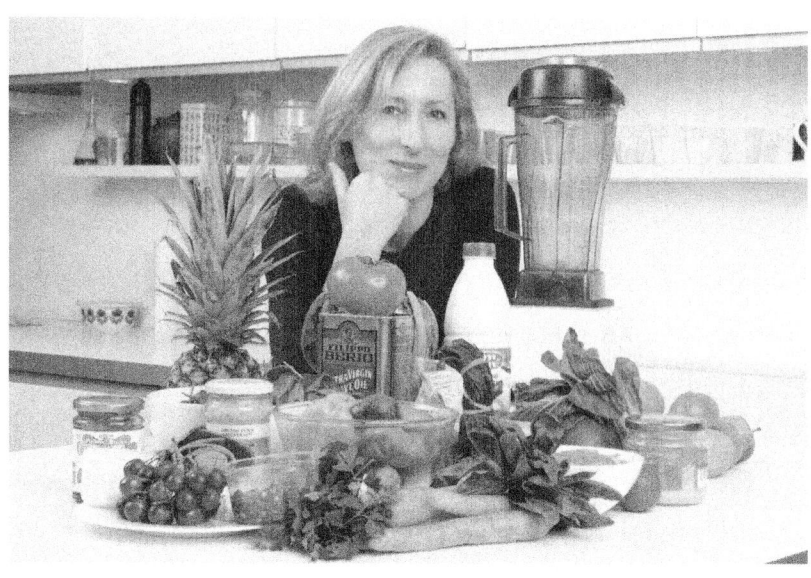

Intermittent Fasting and Longevity

Perhaps the greatest bane of growing older is that old age opens up the body to more risk of developing diseases.

Ultimately, intermittent fasting became so popular among women aged 50 and older because of how it evidently helps them live longer and in good health.

Some even say it was tailor-made for older women.

Intermittent Fasting Boosts Productivity

Intermittent fasting helps you experience a boost in productivity by helping to keep you fit and in good health.

In summary, intermittent fasting is the answer to many of the adverse effects of growing older. It keeps you in charge of your body and teaches you how to get the best out of your body system, effectively maximizing your potential to remain in good health for as long as possible.

Chapter 4. False Myths About IF Diet

There are so many myths about intermittent fasting circulating in health books and on the Internet. These erroneous statements have created a stigma around intermittent fasting that causes people to avoid following this breakthrough diet. Learn to see through these myths which are not true.

Fasting Is Dangerous

This first myth is simply ridiculous. Everyone intermittently fasts as they sleep. Doing it at other times or for a few days on end is no more dangerous than simply fasting while you sleep. The body needs a period to perform autophagy, and it cannot do that if it is too busy processing food all of the time. Intermittent fasting gives your body a well-deserved break while helping you preserve your health.

Remember, fasting is not starvation. You can still eat. Don't confuse fasting, which is healthful with starvation, which is dangerous.

Fasting Can Lower Your Blood Sugar Dangerously

The body can maintain its own blood glucose levels by releasing glycogen, or sugar stored in the liver. This fact means that you won't go low dangerously if you stop eating for a spell. Instead, it will balance out and cause your body to start burning fat. The fat will keep you nourished and prevent fainting from not eating.

If you feel faint or lightheaded, you may need to eat. Be sure to listen to your body. Decrease your fasting period if you keep having dizzy spells.

It Will Cause Hormonal Imbalance

If anything, IF will balance your hormones. Doing IF wrong will indeed cause leptin and ghrelin, the main hunger hormones, to go crazy and make people binge. Then they will feel guilty and restrict themselves more. The hormones will get even more imbalanced. This effect can suppress a woman's ovulation and even stop her period. However, a woman who implements IF correctly by keeping herself nourished in her eating windows will not experience this at all.

It Will Destroy Your Metabolism

Your metabolism will run on whatever energy source is easiest. Sugar from food is the easiest, so your body burns that first. With no sugar present, the body turns to burn its own fat cells. Either way, your metabolism works. You cannot destroy it.

Some say that if you fast, you will overeat and then have even more trouble losing weight. This problem is psychological, not physiological. Often people hate restrictive diets so much that they do overeat when they stop dieting, causing them to gain the weight back. Then, they are resistant to new diet approaches and have trouble losing the regained weight. Affecting over 80% of people who have dieted, this problem is pretty common. But if you stick with IF and nourish yourself properly, you won't return to overeating, and you won't have this problem. IF doesn't ruin your metabolism to the point where you can't lose weight again if you do gain any back.

It Causes Stress

Technically, fasting is a period of stress. But as Dr. Fung points out, it is good stress that causes your cells to do their work more efficiently and handle the stress of illness more successfully. Therefore, fasting will not cause extra stress.

Fasting Can Lead to Overeating

If executed with care, you can avoid the urge to binge eat later. It is true that fasting will make you hungry because of your body's hunger signals. Use bone broth to stave off cravings during fasting periods. Also, avoid going on long fasts when you first start. Don't allow the temptation of food around you or have lots of easy snacks in the house as you fast.

Starvation mode is a myth that some people believe causes the body to hold onto weight when it perceives that it is not getting sufficient calories. Look at any person who has starved themselves, and you will see rapid, immediate weight loss and wasting. That picture of starvation proves that restricting calories to dangerous levels will not cause weight gain, but rather weight loss. Plus, fasting is not a dangerous caloric restriction or starvation so it will not cause any unhealthy "mode."

Fasting Causes the Body to Burn Muscle

Because fasting stimulates the production of HGH, it builds muscle rather than destroys it. It only promotes your body to eat fat, not muscle. People tend to start losing muscle mass if they consume too few calories, or essentially starve themselves. But they will not lose muscle if they stay nourished and hydrated and eat well between fasting periods.

You Can't Work Out While Fasting

You can absolutely work out while fasting. If you have eaten well during your eating window and have some extra body fat, exercise will only make your body burn more. Your body will get the nutrition it needs to fuel the workout from your fat stores and the last meal you ate. Be sure to stay hydrated for energy.

Chapter 5.   Possible Risks of Intermittent Fasting

Even though we can't overlook the way that irregular fasting has a lot of medical advantages. There are significantly more favorable circumstances that are extraordinary for the human body and increment the life expectancy of people too. There are likewise some negative effects of intermittent fasting. Any individual who is going to begin irregular fasting at any point shortly has to know both the positive and negative effects of fasting and afterward choose whether it's advantageous for your body or not.

Getting Started Takes an Adjustment

Any lifestyle change takes an adjustment, and it can take months for something to become a habit. Naturally, intermittent fasting is quite an adjustment for people who are used to grazing on food throughout the day. This means that if you push yourself to go into an advanced version of intermittent fasting when you first begin, you can become overwhelmed. But if you start slowly and allow your body to adjust in its own time, you will find it happens much more naturally and becomes easy to stick to.

Potential to Overeat

While intermittent fasting should naturally reduce caloric intake, if a person pushes themselves to fast when they are overly hungry, it might lead to overeating during their eating window. This is because the person feels hungry for a long time while fasting when they finally eat, their body believes it must make up for the missing calories. The result is that the person either hits a weight loss plateau or even experience increased weight.

Possible Leptin Imbalance

The hormone leptin is important as it signals to your body that you are full have no longer need to eat. But when a person practices intermittent fasting, it may temporarily disrupt this hormone's production. However, this is usually only a short-term problem, and once a person's body adjusts to their fasting and eating windows, their leptin will balance itself out. Typically, a leptin imbalance is only a real problem when a person dives head-first into intermittent fasting and attempt to practice advanced level fasting when they are still only a beginner.

You May Become Dehydrated

Many people do not drink enough water. In general, doctors recommend that we drink half of our body's weight in pounds in ounces of water. This means that if you weigh 200 lbs., you should be drinking one-hundred ounces of water daily.

Lots of people don't drink water that is enough as it's, but this can make dehydration worse when an individual is practicing fasting. This is because fasting boosts the metabolism, and when your cells are in a metabolic accelerated state, they require more water for fuel. If you are not giving them enough water during periods of fasting, you can quickly become dehydrated. Not only that but when fasting, you are likely to lose a lot of water weight, which can result in dehydration and a deficiency in electrolytes. Make sure that you not only drink plenty of water but also consume enough electrolytes to prevent this. Thankfully, dehydration is easy to avoid if you remain proactive.

Not Everyone Can Practice Intermittent Fasting

Intermittent fasting is a beautiful and healthy lifestyle for the general population. After all, the human body is designed for practice periods of fasting naturally. However, not every person can practice fasting. Some people, due to chronic illness, may be unable to participate. Ultimately, you must ask your doctor if you are healthy enough to practice short-term fasting.

It Can Trigger the Re-Feeding Syndrome

This is a hazardous and fatal disorder that can happen if you suffer from malnutrition. It is when electrolyte and liquid imbalances occur when malnourished individuals have been hospitalized for a long time and eat again after a long time. The chance of acquiring re-feeding syndrome increases when bodily weight is very small and not eating for more than ten days.

Having Low Energy

Although after a while starvation passes, life isn't predictable. You can take part in a tiresome activity that makes you hungry and ultimately unproductive until the hunger goes or you eat. You may have been used to eating a bunch of snacks during the day and quit instantly due to fasting, which may cause a few side effects. These side effects involve headaches, bad temper, and lack of power, constipation, and low concentration levels. It may also decrease your motivation. This sort of fasting can have an adverse fitness effect if you have a health condition. It is not suitable for all. For example, hypoglycemic people require glucose all day, so they can't profit from fasting.

Interfere With the Social Side of Eating

Eating from ancient times was a significant social event. Special times, festivities, milestone accomplishments, and other activities require meal sharing with your friends. IF can mess with your personal life when you change your routine which may not correspond to the regular eating schedule. On occasions where everyone eats and eats, you may stand out as the one who does not want to participate. Many activities including dinner meetings, family meals, and romantic meals are missed among many others.

Reproductive Complications in Some Women

If the fasting is carried out in a fashion that mainly restricts carbs and protein, it can trigger fertility problems in females, lead to electrolyte defects, and trigger nutritional deficits. There are also long-term adverse health effects. Intermediate fasting is linked to menstrual, premature menopause, and health problems. Research indicates that ovary size can be reduced, thus influencing reproduction and decreasing bodily volume.

Digestive Complications

It can lead to problems linked to digestion. When food is eaten too rapidly, a large meal may cause digestive problems. People who tend to have larger dishes during the feeding period, require to digest them for a longer period. It increases the pressure on your digestive system, triggering indigestion and bloating. This will have a stronger impact on people with weak guts.

Weight Regains

Intermittent acceleration reduces the body's reliance on carbohydrates for fuel and decreases fat dependency for power. There is an improvement in the decomposition of stored fats. The body undergoes physiological changes as a reaction to a drastic decrease in the body's power consumption. This implies that you might not be in a position to keep the weight of yours or perhaps even gain more weight despite extreme dietary restrictions.

Having seen the strengths and downsides of this fasting protocol, it is evident that each benefit's amount and weight is more advantageous than the downsides. Intermittent fasting will greatly improve the quality and the quantity of your life without a doubt.

Chapter 6. Different Types of IF Diet

There are so many different ways to practice intermittent fasting. I will guide you through different specific and different methods for IF.

16/8 Method

This is just about the most popular fasting method since it's so schedule-based, meaning there are no surprises. This will give you the freedom to control when you eat based on your everyday life. The sixteen is the number of hours you're likely to be fasting, which may also be lowered to twelve or perhaps fourteen hours if that fits into your life better. Then your eating period is going to be between eight and ten hours every day. This might seem daunting, but it just means that you are skipping an entire meal. Many people choose to begin their fast around 7–8 p.m. and then do not eat until 11 or noon the next day, which means they fast for the recommended 16 hours. Of course, it isn't as bad as it sounds since they are sleeping during this time, so what it comes down to is eating dinner and then not eating the next day again around lunch, so you are just skipping breakfast.

You will be doing it every day, so finding the hours that work for you are important. If you work the third shift, then switching you're eating period around to fit into your schedule is important. If you find yourself being run down and sluggish, tweak your fasting hours until you find a healthy balance. Granted, there will be some adjustment because chances are, your body is not accustomed to skipping entire meals.

Lean-Gains Method (14:10)

The lean-gains method has several different incarnations on the web, but its fame comes from the fact that it helps shed fat while building it into muscle almost immediately. Through the lean-gains method, you'll find yourself able to shift all that fat to be muscle through a rigorous practice of fasting, eating right, and exercising.

Through this method, you fast anywhere from 14–16 hours and spend the remaining 10–8 hours each day engaged in eating and exercise. As opposed to the crescendo, this method features daily fasting and eating, rather than alternated days of eating versus not. Therefore, you don't have to be quite cautious about extending the physical effort to exercise on the days you are fasting because those days when you're fasting are every day!

For the lean-gaining method, start fasting only for 14 hours and work it up to 16 if you feel comfortable with it, but never forget to drink enough water and be careful about spending too much energy on exercise! Remember that you want to grow in health and potential through intermittent fasting. You'll certainly not want to lose any of that growth by forcing the process along.

20:4 Method

Stepping things up a notch from the 14:10 and 16:8 methods, the 20:4 method is a tough one to master, for it is rather unforgiving. People talk about this method of intermittent fasting as intense and highly restrictive. Still, they also say that the effects of living this method are almost unparalleled with all other tactics.

For the 20:4 method, you'll fast for 20 hours each day and squeeze all your meals, all your eating, and all your snacking into 4 hours. People who attempt 20:4 normally have two smaller meals or just one large meal and a few snacks during their 4-hour window to eat, and it is up to the individual which four hours of the day they devote to eating.

The trick for this method is to make sure you're not overeating or bingeing during those 4-hour windows to eat. It is all-too-easy to get hungry during the 20-hour fast and have that feeling then propel you into intense and unrealistic hunger or meal sizes after the fast period is over. Be careful if you try this method. If you're new to intermittent fasting, work your way up to this one gradually, and if you're working your way up already, only make the shift to 20:4 when you know you're ready. It would surely disappoint if all your progress with intermittent fasting got hijacked by one poorly thought-out goal with the 20:4 method.

Meal Skipping

Meal skipping is an extremely flexible form of intermittent fasting that can provide all of the benefits of intermittent fasting but with less strict scheduling. If you are not someone who has a typical schedule or feels like a stricter variation of the intermittent fasting diet will serve you, meal skipping is a viable alternative.

Many people who choose to use meal skipping find it a great way to listen to their bodies and follow their basic instincts. If they are not hungry, they simply don't eat that meal. Instead, they wait for the next one. Meal skipping can also help people who have time constraints and who may not always be able to get in a certain meal of the day.

It is important to realize that with meal skipping, you may not always be maintaining a 10–16-hour window of fasting. As a result, you may not get every benefit that comes from other fasting diets. However, this may be a great solution for people who want an intermittent fasting diet that feels more natural. It may also be a great idea for those looking to begin listening to their bodies more so that they can adjust to a more extreme variant of the diet with greater ease. It can be a great transitional diet for you if you are not ready to jump into one of the other fasting diets just yet.

Warrior Diet Fasting

The most extreme form of intermittent fasting is known as the Warrior Diet. This intermittent fasting cycle follows a 20-hour fasting window with a short 4-hour eating window. During that eating window, individuals are supposed only to consume raw fruits and vegetables. They can also eat one large meal. Typically, the eating window occurs at night time, so people can snack throughout the evening, have a large meal, and then resume fasting.

Because of the length of fasting taking place during the Warrior Diet, people should also consume a fairly hearty level of healthy fats. Doing so will give the body something to consume during the fast to produce energy with. Additional carbohydrates are also used to increase energy levels; too.

People who eat the Warrior Diet tend to believe that humans are natural nocturnal eaters and that we are not meant to eat throughout the day. The belief is that eating this way follows our natural circadian rhythms, allowing our body to work optimally.

The only people who should consider doing the Warrior Diet are those who have already had success with other forms of intermittent fasting and who are used to it. Attempting to jump straight into the Warrior Diet can have serious repercussions for anyone who is not used to intermittent fasting. Even still, those who are used to it may find this particular style too extreme for them to maintain.

Eat-Stop-Eat (24 Hour) Method

This method of fasting is incredibly similar to the crescendo method. The only discernable difference is that there's no anticipation of increasing into a more intense fasting pattern with time. For the eat-stop-eat method, you decide which days you want to take off from eating, and then you run with it until you've lost that weight, and then you keep running with the lifestyle for good because you won't be able to imagine life without it.

The eat-stop-eat method involves one to two days a week being 100% oriented towards fasting, with the other five to six days concerning "business as normal." The one or two days spent fasting are then full 24-hour days spent without eating anything at all. These days, of course, water and coffee are still fine to drink, but no food items can be consumed whatsoever. Exercise is also frowned upon on those fasting days but see what your body can handle before you decide how that should all work out.

Some people might start thinking they're using the crescendo method but end up sticking with eat-stop-eat.

Alternate-Day Method

The alternate-day method is admittedly a little confusing, but the reason it could be so confusing could come, in part, from how much wiggle room it provides for the practitioner. This method is great for people who don't have a consistent schedule or any sense of one; it is incredibly forgiving for those who don't quite have everything together for themselves yet.

When it comes down to it, alternate-day intermittent fasting is really up to you. You should try to fast every other day, but it doesn't have to be that precise. Similarly, with the crescendo method, as long as you fast two to three days a week, with a break day or two in between each fasting day, you're set! Then, you'll want to eat normally for three or four days out of each week, and when you encounter a fasting day, you don't even need to completely fast!

Alternate-day fasting is a solid place to start from, especially if you work a varying schedule or still have yet to get used to a consistent one. If you want to make things more intense from this starting point, the alternate-day method can easily become the eat-stop-eat method, the crescendo method, or the 5:2 method. Essentially, this method is a great place to begin

12:12 Method

As another of the more natural ways of intermittent fasting, the 12:12 approach is well-suited to beginning practitioners. Many people live out the 12:12 method without any forethought simply because of their sleeping and eating schedule, but turning 12:12 into a conscious practice can have just as many positive effects on your life as the more drastic 20:4 method claims.

According to a study conducted at the University of Alabama, for this method, in particular, you fast for 12 hours and then enter a 12-hour eating window. It's not difficult whatsoever to get three small meals and several snacks, or two big meals and a snack into your day with this method. With 12:12, the standard meal timing works just fine.

Ultimately, this method is a great one to start from, for a lot of variation can be built into this scheduling when you're ready to make things more interesting. Effortlessly and without much effort, 12:12 can become 14:10 or even 16:8, and in seemingly no time, you can find yourself trying alternate-day or crescendo methods, too. Start with what's normal for you, and this method might be exactly that!

Chapter 7. Practical Support to Fasting

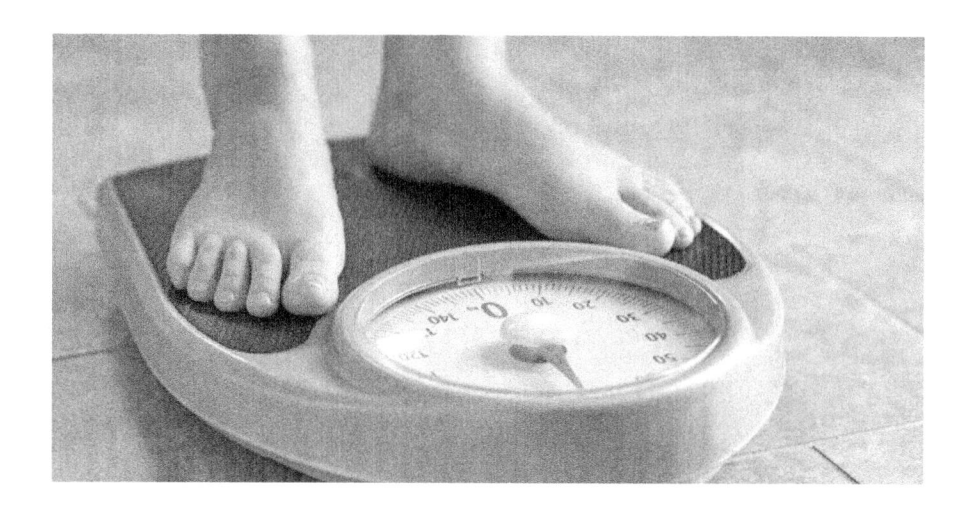

The Mindset for Success

When it comes to fasting, it is important to ensure that you approach it in a way that will be beneficial for our health, and that will not do more harm than good. Firstly, you want to maintain flexibility with yourself and your body when fasting.

For example, if you are not feeling well as you are trying to fast, don't be afraid to eat a small amount on your fast days. This is especially true at the beginning when you first introduce fasting into your diet. If you try a water fast, for example, and you feel lightheaded and weak, you may decide that you want to instead try an intermittent fasting method like 5:2 which would allow you to eat on your fast days, but in a greatly restricted amount. If you have your mindset on the 24-hour water fast, then try the 5:2 method a few times before you try the full water fast in order to get your body comfortable with reduced amounts of food first.

Maintaining this flexible mindset will allow you to remain healthy, and it will allow you to pay more attention to how you are feeling than to the plan that you have set out for yourself.

The Biggest Obstacle: Your Mind

Everybody's objective will differ slightly and will likely be quite personal to them. Maybe you want to reduce your risk of cancer because it runs in your family. Maybe you have been obese for the majority of your life, and you are trying this as a means of weight loss and health improvement. Maybe you heard about it and challenged yourself to try it for a few months to see how it feels. Whatever your objective, writing it down will help to solidify it and make it real. Then, when you are wondering why on earth you decided to put yourself through this on the first day of your fast, you can look at that objective that you wrote down, and it will re-inspire you to continue. When it comes to mindset, being aware of your motivation is extremely beneficial.

When it comes to something like fasting, the mental game is the biggest part of it. You already know that your body can survive without ingesting food for the time that you plan to fast. You know that you will be giving it food at the end of this fasting period. You know that your body will likely even be better for having fasted. What all this means is that the part that makes it very difficult is the mental part. During a fast, the mindset will play a huge part in how you feel.

What you choose to focus on during your fast will determine if you are having a terrible time and counting down the hours until you can eat again, or if you barely notice them going by. By focusing on what you are depriving yourself of you will see everything as a punishment, you are putting yourself through. Instead, if you look at the things that you are giving yourself—like tea, black coffee, and water and appreciate these things, it will help you to rediscover how refreshing and nourishing water is, a fact that we take for granted in places where the water is clean and drinkable. You will be able to taste the coffee beans without the cream and sugar that cover up their beauty. You will be able to appreciate the tea leaves that spend time growing in order to end up in this cup of yours. You will also appreciate your food that much more when you reach your eating window, and you can eat whatever you want. By viewing your day through the lens of appreciation instead of deprivation, you will have a much easier time with your fast.

Set Goals

A healthy weight loss goal is to lose between 1–2 lbs. every week. If you start losing more, there's a chance that you are losing muscle mass. There's credible research to confirm that it's possible to lose lean muscle mass with Intermittent Fasting if you don't eat enough protein. You can be healthy when it comes to weight but still have high amounts of abdominal fat, which can cause many health risks. The goals with Intermittent Fasting depend on your health and weight goals. You can determine your diet goals by answering a couple of simple questions:

Which improvements are you seeking? Do you want to?

- Reduce the symptoms of illness
- Feel better
- Become more energized
- Lose weight
- All of the above?
- Are you interested in practicing the diet long-term, or only until you meet your goals?
- How will you track the intake of macronutrients?
- What are your diet preferences?

Calculate Body Mass Index

Your BMI can be higher if you are masculine, which doesn't mean that you should lose weight if you are healthy. You can think of yourself as obese if your BMI is over 30. However, this isn't exclusive to the number because it's possible to have a healthy weight with an unhealthy amount of body fat. These are rough calculations that can cause you to think of someone who is athletic, as well as someone who is thinner but has as body fat as an obese. However, calculating your BMI can help you determine your goals for weight loss in collaboration with your doctor and a dietitian.

Calculate the Body Fat Percentage

Looking into your body-fat percentage will help you to understand what you should do to lose weight, for example:

- Which method of Intermittent Fasting is the most appropriate?
- Whether or not you want to incorporate the Keto diet in Intermittent Fasting?
- How much do you need to exercise, and what kind of exercises are necessary?

If you like exercising, Intermittent Fasting will help you lose body fat, but preserve or gain muscle mass. As a result, you may not notice scaling down. However, even if you don't lose weight, but gain muscle mass, you will still look slimmer.

To track how your body fat changes, you can use the body composition scales. These scales help you track how your muscle mass, your hydration, and your body fat change throughout your diet.

Calculate Waist-to-Hip Ratio

The waist-hip ratio or WHR is a more credible measurement because it accounts for your natural body shape. For women, an ideal measure is 0.8, while 0.9 is ideal for men. If your measurements are higher, you should work on your shape.

For calculating the WHR, you can use a tape measure and measure the circumference of the widest part of your hips and your natural waist, which is slightly above your belly button. After that, divide your waist measurement by your hip measurement.

Plan Your Portions

Calculate Basal Metabolic Rate

While measuring meals isn't required with Intermittent Fasting, it is desirable to maintain optimal health levels. To start, you should calculate your basal metabolic rate to find out how many calories you need to maintain your weight, and how many you need to lose it.

Calculate the Right Portion Sizes

When calculating portion sizes, keep in mind that 1 gram of nutrients translates to a different number of calories:

- Fat: 9 calories
- Protein: 4 calories
- Carbohydrates: 4 calories

Calculate the Daily Calorie Intake

In general, Intermittent Fasting doesn't require calorie restriction for weight loss. Still, weight loss and other health benefits of fasting will be greater if you have a controlled daily calorie intake.

A Step-by-Step Approach

If you follow a very hard approach from the word GO, you are bound to face adjustment issues. The best approach is to allow the body to adapt to the fasting schedule and let it build the capacity to stay hungry.

Eliminate Snacks

This is something that would come several times in this book. It is a very important thing that you must understand. The root cause of most of our health issues is the habit of frequent snacking.

Snacking leads to 2 major issues:

1. It keeps causing repeated glucose spikes that invoke an insulin response and hence the overall insulin presence in the bloodstream increases aggravating the problem of insulin resistance.
2. It usually involves refined carb and sugar-rich food items that will lead to cravings and you will keep feeling the urge to eat at even shorter intervals.

This is a reason your preparation for intermittent fasting must begin with the elimination of snacks. You can have 2–3 nutrient-dense meals in a day, but you will have to remove the habit of snacking from your routine.

As long as the habit of snacking is there, you'll have a very hard time staying away from food as this habit never allows your ghrelin response clock to get set at fixed intervals. This means that you will keep having urges to eat sweets and carb-rich foods, and you will also have strong hunger pangs at regular intervals.

The farther you can stay away from refined carb-rich and sugar-rich food items, the easier you would find it to deal with hunger.

You Must Start Easy. Don't Do Anything Drastic or Earth-Shattering

Simply start by lowering the number of snacks you have in a day. The snacks have not only become a need of the body, but they are also a part of the habit. In a day, there are numerous instances when we eat tit-bits that we don't care about. We sip cold drinks, sweetened beverages, chips, cookies, bagels, donuts, burgers, pizzas simply because they are in front of us or accessible. We have made food an excuse to take breaks. This habit will have to be broken if you want to move on the path of good health.

Widen the Gap Between Your Meals

This process needs to be gradual and should only begin when you have eliminated snacks from your routine. Two nutrient-dense meals in a day or two meals and a smaller meal or lunch comprising of fiber-rich salads should be your goal.

However, you must remember that these two steps must be taken over a long period. You must allow your body to get used to the change. There would be a temptation that it is easy to follow these, and you can jump to the actual intermittent fasting routine, but it is very important to avoid all such temptations as they are only going to lead to failures.

If your body doesn't get used to this routine, very soon, you'll start feeling trapped. You'll start finding ways to cheat the routine. You'll look for excuses to violate the routine, and it very soon becomes a habit. This is the reason you must allow your body to take some time to adjust to the new schedule.

You should remember that intermittent fasting is a way of life. This might slower the results, but it is going to make your overall journey smoother and better.

The Best Tips and Tricks for Starting Intermittent Fasting

Intermittent fasting is not easy. We need support as much as possible and anything that can make your journey easier. Below are some of the tips that will make your journey smooth and effective.

Decide on Your Fasting Window

Intermittent fasting is not a strict time-based diet. This means that you can choose the number of hours to fast and when to fast either day or night. The fasting and eating window periods are not a must to be the same every day.

Ensure You Get Enough Sleep

When you get enough sleep, you become healthier, and your overall well-being is guaranteed. When we sleep, the body operates certain functions in the body that helps burn calories and improve the metabolic rate.

Eat Healthy Avoid Eating Anything You Want After a Fast

Healthy meals should be your focus. They will help you get the required nutrients like vitamins, which will give you more energy during the fasting period.

Drink More Water

One of the best decisions you can make during a fast is to drink water. It will keep your body hydrated, and taking water before meals can significantly reduce appetite.

Start Small

For beginners, you can start by having your food at 8 pm, for example, and having nothing again until 8 am the next day. It will be easier since sleep is incorporated into your eating window.

Avoid Stress

Intermittent fasting might be hard to do if you are stressed. This is because stress can trigger an overindulgence of food in some people. It is also easier to feed on junk when stressed to feel better. That's why when on intermittent fasting, you are advised to control your stress levels.

Be Disciplined

Remember that fasting means the abstinence of food until a particular time. When fasting, be true to yourself and avoid eating before the stipulated time. It will ensure that you lose maximum weight and benefit health-wise from intermittent fasting.

Keep Yourself Off Flavored Drinks

Most flavored drink says that they are low in sugar, but in the real sense, they are not. Flavored drinks contain artificial sweeteners, which will affect your health negatively. They will also increase your appetite, causing you to overeat, and this will make you gain weight instead of losing.

Exercising

Exercise can be done when fasting, but it is not a must. Mild exercises can be done even at home. By exercising, you will build your muscle strength, and your body fat will burn faster.

Intermittent Fasting and Exercise

The women above fifties have a hard time taking care of their bodies if they aren't active. Our body is unhealthy if it is subjected too long to a sedentary lifestyle. There are multiple reasons for it. Some of the most active women I have seen in their fifties moved around their bodies quite a lot. They exercised their bodies, easily staying fit even when they aged. There were also the cases of women who were only forty-five but they had the problems of sixty-five years old women. I expected as much seeing their sedentary lifestyle. The exercise makes a hell lot of difference.

When you move around your body, you automatically push your body to regulate its functions, performing well. The body needs exercise just as our functions need to perform well. Exercise is the biggest difference-maker. It is that healthy habit that decides if you will automatically have a body of a thirty-year-old while remaining fifty or have a body of a sixty-five-year-old while remaining forty.

Generally, there are two kinds of females. The first type of female includes those ladies who have remained active in their youth. When they were in their twenties or thirties even, they moved around quite a lot. Yoga, jogging, and aerobics are something known to them. Naturally, they are also the women who can do intermittent fasting better. Even if you are a woman in your fifties, you will remain much fitter if you exercised in your prime years.

There is another type of female who has led a sedentary style of life. Those females are often inactive, lacking any interest in exercise or physical activity. Often, the busy routine along with the field of work make this thing possible.

I can give you a piece of good news. Females who have not exercised in their twenties or even thirties can still reap the benefits of exercise. As you do intermittent fasting, you will realize that your bodies are more mobile than before, easily being able to do things you didn't think were possible. Even if you were a female who had led a life of physical inactiveness, you still have a shot at it. Intermittent fasting naturally reduces cholesterol, leading to a mobile and active body.

For the females who had been quite active before and still do a tremendous amount of exercise, I would suggest cutting down a bit. Intermittent fasting combined with exercise is somewhat a powerful combo for weight loss and cholesterol reduction. However, you must avoid exhaustion. I will give a list of the best exercises that are well suited for the women above fifties. You can choose a suitable time for these exercises like in the morning or evening. Make sure to never overexert your body. Your body is your temple and the more you take care of it, the more it will take care of you.

Practical Exercises at Home Without Tools Suitable for Women Over 50 and Instructions on How to Perform Them

You know well that daily exercises help you to achieve a healthy weight. Through physical activity, you help the body to burn fat, to work the areas where it is localized, and, gradually, you tone your body to make it more beautiful.

You don't need to go out all the time for your workout routines; you can do just as much staying indoors. Many workouts don't need either a gym membership or equipment to do.

Yoga

Yoga is good for everyone: men, women, and children, but it is especially excellent for all women. We, women, have precise needs, problems, and stages of life. Just think for a moment about how much a woman's attitude and physical health are affected by hormones, which control the menstrual cycle, pregnancy, and menopause. Yoga balances these hormones efficiently and effectively during the many stages of life.

Yoga, however, is not only for the changes in the body to which women are subjected, but also serves to balance emotions, to reduce the impact of diseases such as breast cancer and osteoporosis, and for the female need to have a way to live comfortable and relaxed, following the spiritual attitude.

Yoga is one of the most straightforward workouts you can do. No matter your abilities and needs, there are many yoga styles designed to meet your needs. Maybe you want to stretch your body or relax, or perhaps you want to calm down, yoga can help you achieve all these.

You can get some props like blocks and straps, but you can replace them with other objects. You can use rolls of paper towels or a stack of books instead as a yoga block for extra lift during poses.

In the most common yoga exercises, you work simultaneously on strength, balance, and stretching. Thanks to the different types of positions practiced, you get these benefits:

- Greater oxygenation of internal organs and tissues, therefore a detox action
- Posture improvement, especially in the case of "alignment focused" practices
- Flexibility and ease of movement
- Muscle toning
- Improved blood circulation
- Breath control and regularization
- Improvement of blood pressure
- Stabilization of blood sugar
- Increase in bone mass
- Improvement of digestive problems
- Stimulation of the parasympathetic nervous system

Plank

Plank is another excellent exercise that doesn't need any equipment. There are many variations you can pick from depending on your goals.

It has become famous worldwide for its effectiveness. This type of exercise is for the abdomen, but at the same time, it works on all the muscles of the body.

To notice the results of this exercise, the only thing you need is a good dose of willpower to put it into practice. It is essential to repeat this exercise every day, at least once a day, for a few minutes. This is not an easy exercise, as it consists of supporting yourself with your hands and feet for several minutes without stopping. By keeping this position, the various muscles are activated, and, as a result, you will get a strong back, fit legs, a flat abdomen, more toned arms, and buttocks.

You can start with the type that involves your knees being bent while on the floor instead of your legs being straight. You may find it easier to bend your elbows and rest your forearms on the floor instead of doing the plank that involves your arms straight with your hands on the floor.

To mix things up, you can try working on different parts of your core by trying a side plank. While lying on your side, place your feet on one of each other. While using an arm to support your weight, push yourself off the floor. Make sure your body is in a straight line and keep you're your front facing out, so your hips are elevated. Try to hold your pose for as long as possible. Face to the other side and try to do the same.

Walking the Stairs

Walking up and down the stairs allows you to improve the health of your heart and lungs, has a low impact on the joint, and is useful for developing speed, power, and agility.

You can train at different degrees of intensity depending on your physical condition. This type of training leads the lower body muscles (thighs, buttocks, and calves) to work hard anyway, as they have to repeatedly lift the upper part of the person in a vertical movement that goes against the force of gravity.

When you go up and down the stairs, with a certain intensity, you burn a high amount of fat more than running and fast walking. This simple activity can also help strengthen the muscles that stabilize the knees, ligaments, and cartilages; in this regard, stairs are often included in rehabilitation activities. It also helps to normalize blood pressure levels and heart health in general. It is an excellent exercise to improve balance, strength, endurance, and sculpt and slim the muscles of the lower body.

Squats and Lunges

Squats and lunges are great for improving your lower body strength. Just like planks, squats and lunges are more complicated than they appear. Squats are ideal exercises when you train at home: they do not require the use of special tools (unless you add weights), they can be performed anywhere with a free body, they are suitable for any time of the day.

But how do you squat? Correct posture is essential both to benefit from the toning effects of the exercise and to avoid incurring tears or painful contractures. So the squat mimics the act of sitting, but without the chair. Although the first few times, perhaps it would be useful to use a chair, obviously without being able to lean on it, merely keeping it as a reference point.

To begin, start by standing up straight, then place your feet apart and look straight in front of you.

For a lunge, stand with your feet only a few inches apart and your eyes staring straight ahead. Step forward with just a leg while lowering your hips slowly towards the ground with your knees bent. The knees of your forward leg should be in line with your ankle instead of just jutting it out. Stay in the lunge position for a beat before going back to standing. Repeat for a few minutes by alternating your legs.

Mistakes to Avoid During Intermittent Fasting Diet

When you are looking to make any significant adjustments in your life, it can take time to discover exactly how to do it in the best ways possible. Many people will make mistakes and have some setbacks as they seek to improve their health through intermittent fasting. Some of these mistakes are minor and can easily be overcome, whereas others may be dangerous and could cause serious repercussions if they are not caught in time.

In this section, we are going to explore common mistakes that people tend to make when they are on the intermittent fasting diet. We will also explore why these mistakes are made, and how they can be avoided. It is important that you read through this chapter before you actually commit to the diet itself. That way, you can ensure that you are avoiding any potential mistakes beforehand. This will help you in avoiding unwanted problems and achieving your results with greater success and fewer setbacks.

Switching Too Fast

A significant number of people fail to comply with their new diets because they attempt to go too hard too fast. Trying to jump too quickly can result in you feeling too extreme of a departure from your normal. As a result, both psychologically and physically you are put under a significant amount of stress from your new diet. This can lead to you feeling like the diet is not actually effective and like you are suffering more than you are actually benefitting from it.

If you are someone who eats regularly and who frequently snacks, switching to the intermittent fasting diet will take time and patience. I cannot stress the importance of your transition period enough.

It is not uncommon to want to jump off the deep end when you are making a lifestyle change. Often, we want to experience great results right away and we are excited about the switch. However, after a few days, it can feel stressful. Because you didn't give your mind and body enough time to adapt to the changes, you ditch your new diet in favor of more comfortable things.

Fasting is something that should always be acclimated to over a period of time. There is no set period, it needs to be done based on what feels right for you and your body. If you are not properly listening to your body and its needs you are going to end up suffering in major ways. Especially with diets like intermittent fasting, letting yourself adapt to the changes and listening to your body's needs can ensure that you are not neglecting your body in favor of strictly following someone else's guide on what to do.

You Are Giving Up Too Quickly

A lot of people assume that eating the intermittent fasting diet means that they will see the benefits of their eating habits immediately. This is not the case. While intermittent fasting does typically offer great results fairly quickly, it does take some time for these results to begin appearing.

You might feel compelled to quickly give up if you do not begin noticing your desired results right away, but trust that this is not going to help you. Some people require several weeks before they really begin seeing the benefits of their dieting. This does not mean that it is not working, it simply means that it has taken them some time to find the right balance so that they can gain their desired results and stay healthy.

A great way to do this is to try using your food diary once again. For a few days, track how you are eating in accordance with the intermittent fasting diet and what it is doing for you. Get a clear idea of how much you are eating, what you are eating, and when you are eating it. Also, track the amount of physical activity that you are doing on a daily basis.

Through tracking your food intake and exercise levels, you might find that you are not experiencing the results you desire because you are eating too much or not enough in comparison to the amount of energy you are spending each day. Then, you can easily work towards adjusting your diet to find a balance that supports you in getting everything you need and also seeing the results that you desire.

In most cases, intermittent fasting diets are not working because they are not being used right for the individual person. Although the general requirements are somewhat the same, each of us has unique needs based on our lifestyles and our unique makeup. If you are willing to invest time in finding the right balance for yourself then you can guarantee that you can overcome this and experience great results from your fasting.

Choosing the Wrong Plan for Your Lifestyle

It is not uncommon to forget the importance of picking a fasting cycle that actually fits with your lifestyle and then fitting it in. Trying to fast to a cycle that does not fit with your lifestyle will ultimately result in you feeling inconvenienced by your diet and struggling to maintain it.

Often, the way we naturally eat is in accordance with what we feel fits into our lifestyle in the best way possible. So, if you look at your present diet and notice that there are a lot of convenience meals and they happen all throughout the day, you can conclude two things: you are busy, and you eat when you can. Picking a diet that allows you to eat when you can is important in helping you stick to it. It is also important that you begin searching for healthier convenience options so that you can get the most out of your diet.

Anytime you make a lifestyle change, such as with your diet, you need to consider what your lifestyle actually is. In an ideal world, you may be able to completely adapt everything to suit your dreamy needs. However, in the real world, there are likely many aspects of your lifestyle that are simply not practical to adjust. Picking a diet that suits your lifestyle rather than picking a lifestyle that suits your diet makes far more sense.

Taking the time to actually document what your present eating habits are like before you embark on your intermittent fasting diet is a great way to begin. Focus on what you are already eating and how often and consider diets that will serve your lifestyle. You should also consider your activity levels and how much food you truly need at certain times of the day. For example, if you have a spin class every morning, fasting until noon might not be a good idea as you could end up hungry and exhausted after your class. Choosing the dieting pattern that fits your lifestyle will help you actually maintain your diet so you can continue receiving great results from it.

Eating Too Much or Not Enough

Focusing on what you are eating and how much you are eating is important. This is one of the biggest reasons why a gradual and intentional transition can be helpful. If you are used to eating throughout the entire day, attempting to eat the same amount in a shorter window can be challenging. You may find yourself feeling stuffed and far too full to actually sustain that amount of eating on a day-to-day basis. As a result, you may find yourself not eating enough.

If you are new to intermittent fasting and you take the leap too quickly, it is not unusual to find yourself scarfing down as much food as you possibly can the moment your eating window opens back up. As a result, you find yourself feeling sick, too full, and uncomfortable. Your body also struggles to process and digest that much food after having been fasting for any given period of time. This can be even harder on your body if you have been using a more intense fast and then you stuff yourself. If you find yourself doing this, it may be a sign that you have transitioned too quickly and that you need to slow down and back off.

You might also find yourself not eating enough. Attempting to eat the same amount that you typically eat in 12–16 hours in just 8–12 hours can be challenging. It may not sound so drastic on paper, but if you are not hungry you may simply not feel like eating. As a result, you may feel compelled to skip meals. This can lead to you not getting enough calories and nutrition on a daily basis. In the end, you find yourself not eating enough and feeling unsatisfied during your fasting windows.

The best way to combat this is to begin practicing making calorie-dense foods before you actually start intermittent fasting. Learning what recipes you can make and how much each meal needs to have in order to help you reach your goals is a great way to get yourself ready and show yourself what it truly takes to succeed. Then, begin gradually shortening your eating window and giving yourself the time to work up to eating enough during those eating windows without overeating. In the end, you will find yourself feeling amazing and not feeling unsatisfied or overeating as you maintain your diet.

Your Food Choices Are Not Healthy Enough

Even if you are eating according to the keto diet or any other dietary style while you are intermittently fasting, it is not uncommon to find yourself eating the wrong food choices. Simply knowing what to eat and what to avoid is not enough. You need to spend some time getting to understand what specific vitamins, and minerals you need to thrive. That way, you can eat a diet that is rich in these specific nutrients. Then, you can trust that your body has everything that it needs to thrive on your diet.

Even though intermittent fasting does not technically outline what you should and should not eat, it is not a one-size-fits-all diet that can help you lose weight while eating anything you want. In other words, excessive amounts of junk foods will still have a negative impact on you, even if you're eating during the right windows.

It is important that you choose a diet that is going to help you maintain everything you need to function optimally. Ideally, you should combine intermittent fasting with another diet such as the keto diet, the Mediterranean diet, or any other diet that supports you in eating healthfully. Following the guidelines of these healthier diets ensures that you are incorporating the proper nutrients into your diet so that you can stay healthy.

Eating the right nutrients is essential as it will support your body in healthy hormonal balances and bodily functions. This is how you can keep your organs functioning effectively so that everything works the way it should. As a result, you end up feeling healthier and experiencing greater benefits from your diet. It is imperative that you focus on this if you want to have success with your intermittent fasting diet.

You Are Not Drinking Enough Fluids

Many people do not realize how much hydration their foods actually give them on a day-to-day basis. Food like fruit and vegetables are filled with hydration that supports your body in healthily functions. If you are not eating as many, then you can guarantee that you are not getting as much hydration as you actually need to be. This means that you need to focus on increasing your hydration levels.

When you are dehydrated you can experience many unwanted symptoms that can make intermittent fasting a challenge. Increased headaches, muscle cramping, and increased hunger are all side effects of dehydration. A great way to combat dehydration is to make sure that you keep water nearby and sip it often. At least once every fifteen minutes to half an hour, you should have a good drink of water. This will ensure that you are getting plenty of freshwater into your system.

Other ways that you can maintain your hydration levels include drinking low-calorie sports drinks, bone broth, tea, and coffee. Essentially, drinking low-calorie drinks throughout the course of the entire day can be extremely helpful in supporting your health. Make sure that you do not exceed your fasting calorie maximum, however, or you will stop gaining the benefits of fasting. As well, water should always be your first choice above any other drinks to maintain your hydration. However, including some of the others from time to time can support you and keep things interesting so that you can stay hydrated but not bored.

If you begin to experience any symptoms of dehydration, make sure that you immediately begin increasing the amount of water that you are drinking. Dehydration can lead to far more serious side effects beyond headaches and muscle cramps if you are not careful. If you find that you are prone to not drinking enough water on a daily basis, consider setting a reminder on your phone that keeps you drinking plenty throughout the day.

The best way to tell that you are staying hydrated enough is to pay attention to how frequently you are peeing. If you are staying in a healthy range of hydration, you should be peeing at least once every single hour. If you aren't, this means that you need to be drinking more water, even if you aren't experiencing any side effects of dehydration. Typically, if you have already begun experiencing side effects then you have waited too long. You want to maintain healthy hydration without waiting for symptoms like headaches and muscle aches to inform you that it is time to start drinking more. This ensures that your body stays happy and healthy and that you are not causing unnecessary suffering or stress to your body throughout the day.

You Are Getting Too Intense or Pushing It

If you are really focused on achieving your desired results, you might feel compelled to push your diet further than what is reasonable for you. For example, attempting to take on too intense of a fasting cycle or trying to do more than your body can reasonably handle. It is not uncommon for people to try and push themselves beyond reasonable measures to achieve their desired results. Unfortunately, this rarely results in them achieving what they actually set out to achieve. It can also have severe consequences.

At the end of the day, listening to your body and paying attention to exactly what it needs is important. You need to be taking care of yourself through proper nutrition and proper exercise levels. You also need to balance these two in a way that serves your body, rather than in a way that leads to you feeling sick and unwell. If you push your body too far, the negative consequences can be severe and long-lasting. In some cases, they may even be life-threatening.

In some cases, pushing your body to a certain extent is necessary. For example, if you are seeking to build more muscle then you want to push yourself to work out enough that your workouts are actually effective. However, if you are pushing yourself to the point that you are beginning to experience negative side effects from your diet, you need to drawback. While certain amounts of side effects are fairly normal early on, experiencing intense side effects, having side effects that don't go away, or having them return is not good. You want to work towards maintaining and minimizing your side effects, not constantly living alongside them. After all, what is the point of adjusting your diet and lifestyle to serve your health if you are not actually feeling healthy while you do it?

Make sure that you check in with yourself on a daily basis to see to it that your physical needs are being met. That way, if anything begins to feel excessive or any symptoms begin to increase, you can focus on minimizing or eliminating them right away. Paying close attention to your needs and looking at your goals long-term rather than trying to reach them immediately is the best way to ensure that you reach your health goals without actually compromising your health while attempting to do so. In the end, you will feel much better about doing it this way.

Chapter 8.   Foods to Eat and Avoid

The main goal of intermittent fasting is to embrace a healthier lifestyle. This means that it should be part of a holistic approach that leads to an overall healthier lifestyle. As such, it's important for you to really take a deep look at what you are eating on non-fast days. In addition, regular exercise and cutting back on harmful substances like cigarettes and alcohol will go a long way toward promoting a host of health benefits.

This is why it's important for you to focus on foods which you should eat and which ones you should. After all, you would only be hurting yourself if you binge on non-fast days and then suddenly flip off the switch on fast days. The gains which you could make in a few weeks of intermittent fasting can be derailed by a couple of binge sessions.

So, let's take a look at foods which you should embrace and the ones which you shouldn't. Ideally, this will become part of your healthier lifestyle plan.

Foods to Embrace

Ideally, intermittent fasting will become part of an overall healthy lifestyle for you. This means that you would be cutting out certain foods that are rather harmful (in excess, of course) and embracing foods that are healthy.

Now, it should be said that during non-fasting days, there are no restrictions on what you can eat. That's why the ideal way to go is to reduce your consumption of foods high in carbs and sugar while embracing fresh foods and lean meats. So, let's take a look at the foods which you ought to make mainstays of your regular diet:

- **Fresh fruits.** The best kind would be fresh without any additives or extra sugar.
- **Raw vegetables.** Nothing frozen. The fresher the better, and they conserve their nutrients much better. Additionally, these can be cooked and consumed on a regular basis.
- **Lean meat.** There are no restrictions on the type of meat you can eat. However, meat that's too fatty may elevate your cholesterol to unhealthy levels.
- **Whole grains.** This is the best way to consume your favorite foods. Whole grains are loaded with fiber while also reducing the number of carbs you consume. Carbs from vegetables and whole grains are far more digestible by the body and lead to less accumulation of fat in the body.
- **Nuts.** Nuts are a good source of healthy fats and protein. They are great during ramp-up and ramp-down times. So, definitely incorporate them into your diet.

As we have mentioned before, the intermittent fasting approach does not openly restrict any foods. So, it's a question of limiting the amount of white, starchy foods and sugar while increasing the number of fresh foods, lean meats, whole grains, and nuts that you consume. When you do this, you give your body the chance to work with quality materials during its repair process.

Foods to Avoid

You often hear health experts demonizing sugar and carbs. Now, it should be said that sugar and carbs are not necessarily bad. They become a problem when they are consumed in excess. When you eat too many of these foods, your body has to play catchup. Naturally, this is where you accumulate fat, gain weight, and see the negative effects of an unhealthy diet.

So, the intermittent fasting approach calls for you to avoid, or at least significantly reduce, the following foods:

- **White starchy foods.** This includes past and potatoes. Starch is metabolized as glucose and immediately goes into fat stores.
- **Foods loaded with carbs.** White bread, or anything baked, is usually loaded with a high amount of carbs.
- **Greasy foods.** Deep-fried and very greasy foods, while tasty, are high in unhealthy fats. These types of fats lead

to high cholesterol. These foods are enemy number one for blood vessel health. They generally lead to poor circulation.

- **Salty foods.** There's nothing wrong with salt unless you eat too much of it. Salting foods to taste is fine. However, excessively salty foods are not only addictive, but they affect your blood pressure and heart health. It's best to switch to sea salt as it contains less sodium.

- **Sugary drinks and alcohol.** By "sugary," we mean things like sodas and iced teas. These are loaded with sugar and other chemicals. Also, alcoholic beverages end up accumulating fat in a heartbeat. Now, consuming moderate amounts of alcohol is perfectly fine (1–2 drinks per week). In fact, a glass of wine will do a great number to your heart. However, it's excessive alcohol consumption that leads to increased fat gains. The reasoning behind this is that alcohol is metabolized by the body the same way sugar is. So, this implies you'll be packing on extra glucose in your system.

Unfortunately, many folks out there go through their entire lives not knowing they are, in fact, allergic to certain foods. For instance, there are folks who are lactose intolerant but don't know it. Other common food allergies are gluten and corn. In particular, corn allergies can lead to quite a bit of digestive distress and inflammation. This is important to note as many of the foods we consume have corn in them.

Lastly, maintaining a healthy diet is all about exercising moderation and common sense. If you are aware of what foods you should cut down on, then it's best to do so. This means that you would be able to enjoy your favorites without too much guilt. However, if you overdo it, then you will find that you can easily derail the hard work you have put in.

So, please keep in mind that maintaining a balanced diet, as much as possible, in tandem with regular exercise, will make intermittent fasting work very well, thereby producing the results you seek.

Chapter 9. How to Practice IF While on Vacation and While Travelling

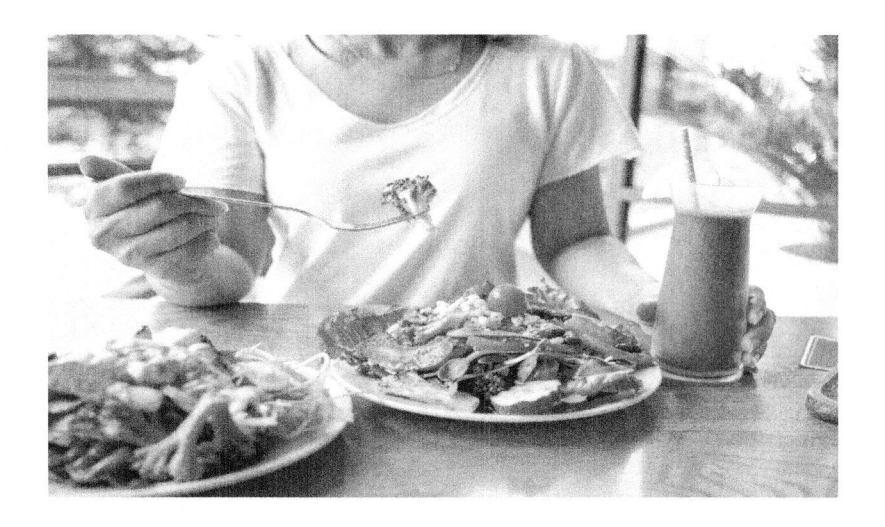

Nutrition Plan

Track your nutritional intake while at home. You must be aware of the number of calories that you consume, the size of the portions, and the composition of your meals. For instance, if you consume 1800 calories in three meals, your dinner can make up for 700 calories, lunch for 400 calories, and the rest for another meal. It means that you can have about 70 g. of protein for lunch and dinner and about 40 g. in another meal.

Stick to the Same Foods

Once you establish your calculated nutrition plan, it is all about sticking to it as much as you can while eating out. Ideally, you must try to stick to similar foods to those that you eat while at home. For instance, if you are used to a meal of meats and vegetables, then order something similar when you go out for a meal. If you go out for a meal, stick to the protein and fibers you eat at home and skip any carb and sugar-rich foods.

Carbs

You need to be careful about the number of carbs you consume. If the dish you ordered has more carbohydrates than you are used to consuming, then simply skip the carbs. Carbs will fill you up for a while and then you will feel hungry again. Instead, fill up on the foods that are good for you. If there is a bread basket on the table, please resist the urge of reaching for it.

Post Meal Hunger

If you want to have a dessert or still have the urge to eat more, even though you are aware that it will exceed your ideal calorie intake, then you need to know that this feeling of hunger will subside soon. A simple trick is to have a cup of tea after a meal, it will make you feel full. It takes about 20 minutes for your brain to signal to you that you are full, so don't keep stuffing yourself with food.

If you follow these simple steps, you can stick to your diet even when you go out for a meal.

Chapter 10. The Combination of IF and Keto Diet

Intermittent fasting and the ketogenic diet are often combined to produce stunning fat loss results. The thing about both ways of eating is that they restrict food in such a way that they promote ketosis or fat burning. They both offer similar health benefits, as well. If used together, they can result in significant fat loss.

How to Combine the Two

Combining keto and fasting is easy. The two methods of eating can work in harmony, turning your body into a sleek fat-burning machine. You pick a fasting plan that works for you from earlier in the book, and then you eat keto-friendly foods on your eating days or during your eating windows.

Possibly the best fasting plan while on keto is the 16:8 method or the 5:2 method. You don't need to go on long fasts while also on keto since your body is already in ketosis from the keto diet plan.

You can use intermittent fasting to reach ketosis first before launching a keto diet. Cleanse your body on a fast, such as the warrior method. When you stop fasting, make sure your meals are ketogenic. You want your first meal to have lots of fat and then continue eating that way. Satiate cravings and prevent overeating during eating windows with low-carb snacks, such as almonds or carrots. Then work fasting into a cycle, balanced with days of keto eating. If you ever slip up on keto by eating too many carbs and leaving ketosis, you can get back into it by fasting for a few days again.

Before you begin this combination, find a keto calculator online for free and enter the appropriate information. You will learn how many carbohydrates, fats, proteins, and overall calories you need per day. You also want to factor in dietary fiber, which keto often neglects to mention. Most people should aim for 25–30 grams of fiber per day. Fiber is essential for your health and smooth, easy stools, which can become too fluid with the high-fat content of ketogenic foods. Fiber has carbs, but they are generally negligible and will not add to your carb allotment.

Benefits of the Keto Diet When You're Fasting

The main benefit of fasting on the keto diet is that you will accelerate results because you will enter ketosis faster. On the keto diet, you restrict carbs and focus on eating high-fat foods to make your body stop relying on sugar and burn fat instead. The presence of ketones in the blood or urine announces that ketosis has commenced. But it can take days and very stringent dietary control to enter ketosis on the keto diet. Since IF can trigger ketosis in a matter of days, versus weeks on ketosis, it allows for entering fat-burning mode more efficiently.

Plus, many people will find themselves out of ketosis if they slip even a tiny bit on their keto diet. A few too many blueberries or a single piece of toast can end ketosis, and then the person must start all over again to get back into it. Fasting when you slip up on keto can help you slide into ketosis again more rapidly.

The diet is simplified with a routine set by fasting, as well. You know exactly what you can eat and when. During your eating window, you should get your calculated rate of fat and protein macros and keep carbs under 20 grams per day. During fasting, you don't have to worry about what to eat at all. And yes, water and bone broth are highly useful on both keto and fasting so that you can use them throughout your diet.

The final and biggest benefit is that IF teaches you not to overeat and overcome cravings. Thus, it prepares your mind for the effort required to stick to the keto eating plan. It also enables you to ignore cravings and control your portions, staying within your macro limits on keto.

Chapter 11. Recipes

Breakfast Recipes

1. Sausage Styled Rolled Omelet

Preparation time: 5 minutes
Cooking time: 8 minutes
Servings: 2

Ingredients

- 1 tbsp. chopped spinach
- 1 tbsp. whipped topping
- 2 eggs
- 2 oz. ground turkey
- 1 tbsp. grated mozzarella cheese

Directions

1. Bring out a skillet pan, put it over medium heat, add ground turkey and cook for 5 minutes until cooked through.
2. Meanwhile, crack eggs in a bowl, add whipped topping and spinach and whisk until combined.
3. When the meat is cooked, put it on a plate, then switch heat to the low level and pour in the egg mixture.
4. Cook the eggs for 3 minutes until the bottom is firm, then flip it and cook for 3 minutes until the omelet is firmed, covering the pan.
5. Sprinkle cheese on the omelet, cook for 1 minute until cheese has melted, and then slide the omelet to a plate.
6. Spread ground meat on the omelet, roll it, then cut it in half and serve.

Nutrition

- Calories: 126
- Carbohydrates: 1 g.
- Fats: 9 g.
- Protein: 10 g.

2. Power Cream With Strawberry

Preparation time: 5 minutes
Cooking time: 0 minutes
Servings: 2

Ingredients

- 1 tbsp. coconut oil
- 1 tsp. vanilla extract, unsweetened
- 2 oz. coconut cream, full-fat
- 2 oz. fresh strawberries

Directions

1. Bring out a large bowl, put all the ingredients in it and then mix by using a blender until smooth.
2. Distribute evenly between two bowls and then serve.

Nutrition

- Calories: 214
- Carbohydrates: 2 g.
- Fats: 3 g.
- Protein: 4 g.

3. Savory Intermittent Pancake

Preparation time: 5 minutes
Cooking time: 5 minutes
Servings: 2

Ingredients

- ¼ cup almond flour
- ½ tbsp. unsalted butter
- 2 eggs
- 1 oz. cream cheese, softened

Directions

1. Bring out a bowl, crack eggs in it, whisk well until fluffy, and then

whisk in flour and cream cheese until well combined.
2. Bring out a skillet pan, put it over medium heat, add butter and when it melts, drop pancake batter in four sections, spread it evenly, and cook for 2 minutes per side until brown.

Nutrition

- Calories: 167
- Carbohydrates: 1 g.
- Fats: 15 g.
- Protein: 2 g.

4. Spinach and Eggs Mix

Preparation time: 5 minutes
Cooking time: 20 minutes
Servings: 4

Ingredients

- 2 tbsp. olive oil
- ½ tsp. smoked paprika
- 12 eggs, whisked
- 2 cups baby spinach
- Salt and black pepper to the taste

Directions

1. Combine all ingredients in a bowl except the oil and whisk them well.
2. Heat up your air fryer at 360°F, add the oil, heat it up, add the eggs and spinach mix, cover, cook for 20 minutes, divide between plates and serve.

Nutrition

- Calories: 220
- Carbohydrates: 4 g.
- Fat: 11 g.
- Fiber: 3 g.
- Protein: 6 g.

5. Savory Ham and Cheese Waffles

Preparation time: 10 minutes
Cooking time: 10 minutes
Servings: 2

Ingredients

- 2 oz. (57 g.) ham steak, chopped
- 2 oz. (57 g.) cheddar cheese, grated
- 8 eggs
- 1 tsp. baking powder
- Basil, to taste

From the cupboard:

- 12 tbsp. butter, melted
- Olive oil, as needed
- 1 tsp. sea salt

Special equipment:

- A waffle iron

Directions

1. Preheat the waffle iron and set it aside.
2. Crack the eggs and keep the egg yolks and egg whites in two separate bowls.
3. Add the butter, baking powder, basil, and salt to the egg yolks. Whisk well. Fold in the chopped ham and stir until well combined. Set aside.
4. Lightly season the egg whites with salt and beat until it forms stiff peaks.
5. Add the egg whites into the bowl of the egg yolk mixture. Allow sitting for about 5 minutes.
6. Lightly coat the waffle iron with olive oil. Slowly pour half of the mixture into the waffle iron and cook for about 4 minutes. Repeat with the remaining egg mixture.
7. Take off from the waffle iron and serve warm on two serving plates.

Nutrition

- Calories: 636

- Fat: 50.2 g.
- Net carbs: 1.1 g.
- Protein: 45.1 g.

6. Classic Spanakopita Frittata

Preparation time: 10 minutes
Cooking time: 3–4 hours
Servings: 8

Ingredients

- 12 eggs, beaten
- ½ cup feta cheese
- 1 cup heavy whipping cream
- 2 cups spinach, chopped
- 2 tsp. garlic, minced

From the cupboard:

- 2 tbsp. extra-virgin olive oil

Directions

1. Grease the bottom of the slow cooker pot with olive oil lightly.
2. Stir together the beaten eggs, feta cheese, heavy cream, spinach, and garlic until well combined.
3. Slowly pour the mixture into the slow cooker. Cook covered on "Low" for 3–4 hours, or until a knife inserted in the center comes out clean.
4. Take off from the slow cooker and cool for about 3 minutes before slicing.
5. Serve and enjoy!

Nutrition

- Calories: 254
- Cholesterol: 364 mg.
- Fat: 22.3 g.
- Fiber: 0 g.
- Net carbs: 2.1 g.
- Protein: 11.1 g.

7. Sausage-Stuffed Bell Peppers

Preparation time: 15 minutes
Cooking time: 4–5 hours
Servings: 4

Ingredients

- 1 cup breakfast sausage, crumbled
- 4 bell peppers, seedless and cut the top
- ½ cup coconut milk
- 6 eggs
- 1 cup cheddar cheese, shredded

From the cupboard:

- 1 tbsp. extra-virgin olive oil
- ½ tsp. freshly ground black pepper

Directions

1. Add the coconut milk, eggs, and black pepper in a medium bowl, whisking until smooth. Set aside.
2. Line your slow cooker insert with aluminum foil. Grease the aluminum foil with 1 tbsp. olive oil.
3. Evenly stuff four bell peppers with the crumbled sausage, and spoon the egg mixture into the peppers.
4. Arrange the stuffed peppers in the slow cooker. Sprinkle the cheese on top.
5. Cook covered on "Low" for 4–5 hours, or until the peppers are browned and the eggs are completely set.
6. Divide among 4 serving plates and serve warm.

Nutrition

- Calories: 459
- Cholesterol: 376 mg.
- Fat: 36.3 g.
- Fiber: 3 g.
- Net carbs: 7.9 g.
- Protein: 25.2 g.

8. Intermittent Tacos With Guacamole and Bacon

Preparation time: 5 minutes
Cooking time: 10 minutes
Servings: 2

Ingredients

- ¼ cup organic Romaine lettuce, chopped
- 3 tbsp. organic sweet potatoes, diced and cooked
- 1 tbsp. Brain Octane oil
- 1 tbsp. ghee, grass-fed
- 2 pieces of eggs, pasture-raised
- 1 piece medium avocado, organic
- 3 slices pastured bacon, cooked
- ¼ tsp. Himalayan pink salt
- Organic micro cilantro (for garnish), as desired

Directions

1. In a skillet over medium heat, heat up the ghee.
2. Get an egg. Crack the egg in the middle of the skillet. Poke the egg yolk.
3. Let the egg cook until solid for about 2 minutes per side. Transfer the cooked egg onto a plate lined with paper towels to absorb the excess oil.
4. Cook the other egg in a similar way. The 2 cooked eggs will serve as the taco shells.
5. In a mixing bowl, put in the avocado, pink salt, and octane oil. Mash the avocado and mix well.
6. Equally, divide the avocado mixture into 2 portions. Spread each avocado mixture onto each egg taco.
7. Arrange the romaine lettuce on top of each taco shell.
8. Put a bacon slice on each taco. Top each taco with the cooked sweet potatoes.
9. Garnish the tacos with micro cilantro and sprinkle some pink salt for added taste.
10. Fold each taco in half. Serve.

Nutrition

- Calories: 387
- Carbs: 9 g.
- Fats: 35 g.
- Fiber: 5 g.
- Proteins: 11 g.

9. Zucchini Pancakes

Preparation time: 5 minutes
Cooking time: 10 minutes
Servings: 3

Ingredients

- 1 ½ oz. zucchini
- ½ cup almond flour
- 2 tbsp. coconut flour
- 2 oz. full-fat milk
- 3 eggs
- ½ tsp. baking powder
- 1 tsp. cinnamon
- 1 tbsp. ghee butter
- Salt and erythritol to taste

Directions

1. Grate the zucchini, season with salt, and place into a sieve to drain
2. Put into a blender, add other ingredients, pulse well
3. Heat then melt the butter in a pan in medium heat
4. Form the pancakes and put them into the skillet
5. Close the lid and cook for 3 minutes on each side

Nutrition

- Calories: 130
- Carbs: 0.7 g.
- Fats: 7 g.
- Protein: 7.5 g.

10. Shrimp Omelet

Preparation time: 5 minutes
Cooking time: 15 minutes
Servings: 4

Ingredients

- 10 oz. boiled shrimps
- 12 eggs
- 4 tbsp. ghee butter
- 4 garlic cloves
- 1 cup intermittent mayo
- 1 fresh red chili peppers
- 1 tbsp. olive oil
- 1 tsp. cumin powder

Directions

1. Mince the garlic cloves and chili pepper
2. In a bowl, blend the shrimps with the mayo, olive oil, minced chili pepper, cumin, minced garlic, salt, and pepper. Set aside for a while
3. In the other bowl, whisk the eggs then add salt and pepper
4. Heat the ghee butter in the skillet, add eggs and shrimp mixture
5. Cook for 5–6 minutes, serve hot

Nutrition

- Calories: 855
- Carbs: 4 g.
- Fat: 82 g.
- Protein: 27 g.

11. Bacon and Zucchini Egg Breakfast

Preparation time: 10 minutes
Cooking time: 10 minutes
Servings: 2

Ingredients

- 2 cups zucchini noodles
- 2 slices of raw bacon
- ¼ cup grated Asiago cheese
- 2 eggs
- Salt and pepper to taste

Directions

1. Cut the bacon slices into ¼-inch thick strips.
2. Cook the bacon in a pan for 3 minutes.
3. Add the zucchini and mix well.
4. Season with salt and pepper.
5. Flatten slightly with a spatula and make 2 depressions for the eggs.
6. Sprinkle with the cheese.
7. Break one egg into each dent.
8. Cook 3 minutes more, then cover and cook for 2–4 minutes, or until the eggs are cooked.
9. Serve.

Nutrition

- Calories: 242
- Fat: 19 g.
- Carb: 4 g.
- Protein: 14 g.

12. Chia Breakfast Bowl

Preparation time: 10 minutes
Cooking time: 0 minutes
Servings: 2

Ingredients

- ¼ cup whole chia seeds
- 2 cups almond milk, unsweetened
- 2 tbsp. sugar-free maple syrup
- 1 tsp. vanilla extract

For the toppings:

- Cinnamon and extra maple syrup, as desired
- Nuts and berries, as desired

Directions

1. Combine the syrup, milk, chia seeds, and vanilla extract in a bowl and stir to mix.
2. Let stand for 30 minutes, then whisk.
3. Transfer to an airtight container.
4. Cover and refrigerate overnight.
5. Serve in the morning.

Nutrition

- Calories: 298
- Fat: 15 g.
- Carb: 5 g.
- Protein: 14 g.

Lunch Recipes

13. Parmesan Roasted Cabbage

Preparation time: 5 minutes
Cooking time: 20 minutes
Servings: 4

Ingredients

- 1 large head green cabbage
- 4 tbsp. melted butter
- 1 tsp. garlic powder
- Salt and black pepper to taste
- 1 cup grated Parmesan cheese
- Grated Parmesan cheese for topping, as desired
- 1 tbsp. chopped parsley to garnish

Directions

1. Set the oven to 400°F, line a baking sheet using foil, and grease with cooking spray.
2. Stand the cabbage and run a knife from the top to bottom to cut the cabbage into wedges. Remove stems and wilted leaves. Mix the butter, garlic, salt, and black pepper until evenly combined.
3. Brush the mixture on every side of the cabbage wedges and sprinkle with Parmesan cheese.
4. Put on the baking sheet, then bake for at least 20 minutes to soften the cabbage and melt the cheese. Remove the cabbages when golden brown, plate, and sprinkle with extra cheese and parsley. Serve warm with pan-glazed tofu.

Nutrition

- Calories: 268
- Fat: 19.3 g.
- Net carbs: 4 g.
- Protein 17.5 g.

14. Briam With Tomato Sauce

Preparation time: 10 minutes
Cooking time: 70 minutes
Servings: 4

Ingredients

- 3 tbsp. olive oil
- 1 large eggplant, halved and sliced
- 1 large onion, thinly sliced
- 3 cloves garlic, sliced
- 5 tomatoes, diced
- 3 rutabagas, diced
- 1 cup sugar-free tomato sauce
- 4 zucchinis, sliced
- ¼ cup water
- Salt and black pepper to taste
- 1 tbsp. dried oregano
- 2 tbsp. chopped parsley

Directions

1. Preheat the oven to 400°F. Warm the olive oil in a skillet at medium heat and cook the eggplant for 6 minutes until on the edges. After, remove to a medium bowl. Sauté the onion and garlic in the oil for 3 minutes and add them to the eggplants. Turn the heat off.
2. In the eggplant bowl, mix in the tomatoes, rutabagas, tomato sauce, and zucchinis. Add the water and stir in the salt, black pepper, oregano, and parsley. Pour the mixture into the casserole dish. Place the dish in the oven and bake for 45–60 minutes. Serve the briam warm on a bed of cauliflower rice.

Nutrition

- Calories: 365
- Fat: 12 g.
- Net carbs: 12.5 g.
- Protein: 11.3 g.

15. Oven-Roasted Cabbage Wedges

Preparation time: 15 minutes
Cooking time: 45 minutes
Servings: 4

Ingredients

- 1 head green cabbage
- ¼ cup olive oil
- 1 ½- tsp. garlic salt
- 1 tsp. onion powder
- 1 tsp. fennel seeds
- ¼ tsp. black pepper

Directions

1. Preheat the stove to 400°F. Line a rimmed heating sheet with a silicone preparing mat or material paper.
2. Cut the cabbage in 1" cuts from one side to the other.
3. Line up the cuts in a solitary layer on a preparing sheet. Brush each wedge with a liberal covering of olive oil.
4. In a little bowl, consolidate garlic salt, onion powder, fennel seeds, and dark pepper. Sprinkle flavoring over each wedge.
5. Prepare for 45 minutes on the center rack—flipping part of the way through.

Nutrition

- Calories: 120
- Carbs: 2.8 g.
- Fat: 9 g.
- Protein: 2 g.

16. Sprouts Stir-Fry With Kale, Broccoli, and Beef

Preparation time: 5 minutes
Cooking time: 8 minutes
Servings: 2

Ingredients

- 3 slices of beef roast, chopped
- 2 oz. Brussels sprouts, halved
- 4 oz. broccoli florets
- 3 oz. kale
- 1 ½ tbsp. butter, unsalted
- ⅛ tsp. red pepper flakes

For the seasoning:

- ¼ tsp. garlic powder
- ¼ tsp. salt
- ⅛ tsp. ground black pepper

Directions

1. Take a medium skillet pan, place it over medium heat, add ¾ tbsp. butter and when it melts, add broccoli florets and sprouts, sprinkle with garlic powder, and cook for 2 minutes.
2. Season vegetables with salt and red pepper flakes, add chopped beef, stir until mixed and continue cooking for 3 minutes until browned on one side.
3. Then add kale along with the remaining butter, flip the vegetables and cook for 2 minutes until kale leaves wilts.
4. Serve.

Nutrition

- Calories: 125
- Fat: 9.4 g.
- Protein: 4.8 g.
- Net carb: 1.7 g.
- Fiber: 2.6 g.

17. Beef and Vegetable Skillet

Preparation time: 5 minutes
Cooking time: 15 minutes
Servings: 2

Ingredients

- 3 oz. spinach, chopped
- ½ lb. ground beef
- 2 slices of bacon, diced
- 2 oz. chopped asparagus
- 3 tbsp. coconut oil
- 2 tsp. dried thyme
- ⅔ tsp. salt

- ½ tsp. ground black pepper

Directions

1. Take a skillet pan, place it over medium heat, add oil and when hot, add beef and bacon and cook for 5–7 minutes until slightly browned.
2. Then add asparagus and spinach, sprinkle with thyme, stir well and cook for 7–10 minutes until thoroughly cooked.
3. Season skillet with salt and black pepper and serve.

Nutrition

- Calories: 332.5
- Fat: 26 g.
- Protein: 23.5 g.
- Net carb: 1.5 g.
- Fiber: 1 g.

18. Beef, Pepper, and Green Beans Stir-Fry

Preparation time: 5 minutes
Cooking time: 18 minutes
Servings: 2

Ingredients

- 6 oz. ground beef
- 2 oz. chopped green bell pepper
- 4 oz. green beans
- 3 tbsp. grated cheddar cheese
- ½ tsp. salt
- ¼ tsp. ground black pepper
- ¼ tsp. paprika

Directions

1. Take a skillet pan, place it over medium heat, add ground beef and cook for 4 minutes until slightly browned.
2. Then add bell pepper and green beans, season with salt, paprika, and black pepper, stir well and continue cooking for 7–10 minutes until beef and vegetables have cooked through.
3. Sprinkle cheddar cheese on top, then transfer pan under the broiler and cook for 2 minutes until cheese has melted and the top is golden brown. Serve.

Nutrition

- Calories: 282.5
- Fat: 17.6 g.
- Protein: 26.1 g.
- Net carb: 2.9 g.
- Fiber: 2.1 g.

19. Cheesy Meatloaf

Preparation time: 5 minutes
Cooking time: 4 minutes
Servings: 2

Ingredients

- 4 oz. ground turkey
- 1 egg
- 1 tbsp. grated mozzarella cheese
- ¼ tsp. Italian seasoning
- ½ tbsp. soy sauce
- ¼ tsp. salt
- ⅛ tsp. ground black pepper

Directions

1. Take a bowl, place all the ingredients in it, and stir until mixed.
2. Take a heatproof mug, spoon in the prepared mixture, and microwave for 3 minutes at high heat setting until cooked.
3. When done, let the meatloaf rest in the mug for 1 minute, then take it out, cut it into two slices and serve.

Nutrition

- Calories: 196.5
- Fat: 13.5 g.
- Protein: 18.7 g.
- Net carb: 18.7 g.
- Fiber: 0 g.

20. Lovely Pulled Chicken Egg Bites

Preparation time: 15 minutes
Cooking time: 30 minutes
Servings: 4

Ingredients

- 2 tbsp. butter
- 1 chicken breast
- 2 tbsp. chopped green onions
- ½ tsp. red chili flakes
- 12 eggs
- ¼ cup grated Monterey Jack

Directions

1. Preheat oven to 400°F. Line a 12-hole muffin tin with cupcake liners. Melt butter in a skillet over medium heat and cook the chicken until brown on each side, 10 minutes.
2. Transfer to a plate and shred with 2 forks. Divide between muffin holes along with green onions and red chili flakes.
3. Crack an egg into each muffin hole and scatter the cheese on top. Bake for 15 minutes until eggs set. Serve.

Nutrition

- Calories: 393
- Fat: 27 g.
- Net carbs: 0.5 g.
- Protein: 34 g.

21. Creamy Mustard Chicken With Shirataki

Preparation time: 20 minutes
Cooking time: 30 minutes
Servings: 4

Ingredients

- 2 (8 oz.) packs of angel hair shirataki
- 4 chicken breasts, cut into strips
- 1 cup chopped mustard greens
- 1 yellow bell pepper, sliced
- 1 tbsp. olive oil
- 1 yellow onion, finely sliced
- 1 garlic clove, minced
- 1 tbsp. wholegrain mustard
- 5 tbsp. heavy cream
- 1 tbsp. chopped parsley

Directions

1. Boil 2 cups of water in a medium pot.
2. Strain the shirataki pasta and rinse well under hot running water. Allow proper draining and pour the shirataki pasta into the boiling water.
3. Cook for 3 minutes and strain again. Place a dry skillet and stir-fry the shirataki pasta until visibly dry, 1–2 minutes; set aside.
4. Heat olive oil in a skillet, season the chicken with salt and pepper, and cook for 8–10 minutes; set aside. Stir in onion, bell pepper, and garlic and cook until softened, 5 minutes.
5. Mix in mustard and heavy cream; simmer for 2 minutes and mix in the chicken and mustard greens for 2 minutes. Stir in shirataki pasta, garnish with parsley and serve.

Nutrition

- Calories: 692
- Net carbs: 15 g.
- Fat: 38 g.
- Protein: 65 g.

22. Parsnip and Bacon Chicken Bake

Preparation time: 10 minutes
Cooking time: 50 minutes
Servings: 4

Ingredients

- 6 bacon slices, chopped
- 2 tbsp. butter
- ½ lb. parsnips, diced

- 2 tbsp. olive oil
- 1 lb. ground chicken
- 2 tbsp. butter
- 1 cup heavy cream
- 2 oz. cream cheese, softened
- 1 ¼ cups grated Pepper Jack
- ¼ cup chopped scallions

Directions

1. Preheat oven to 300°F. Put the bacon in a pot and fry it until brown and crispy, 6 minutes; set aside. Melt butter in a skillet and sauté parsnips until softened and lightly browned. Transfer to a greased baking sheet.
2. Heat olive oil in the same pan and cook the chicken until no longer pink, 8 minutes. Spoon onto a plate and set aside too.
3. Add heavy cream, cream cheese, and two-thirds of the Pepper Jack cheese to the pot. Melt the ingredients over medium heat, frequently stirring, for 7 minutes.
4. Spread the parsnips on the baking dish, top with chicken, pour the heavy cream mixture over, and scatter bacon and scallions.
5. Sprinkle the remaining cheese on top and bake until the cheese melts and is golden, 30 minutes. Serve warm.

Nutrition

- Calories: 757
- Fat: 66 g.
- Net carbs: 5.5 g.
- Protein: 29 g.

23. Blackened Fish With Zucchini Noodles

Preparation time: 10 minutes
Cooking time: 12 minutes
Servings: 2

Ingredients

- 1 large zucchini
- 2 fillets of mahi-mahi
- 1 tsp. Cajun seasoning
- 2 tbsp. butter, unsalted
- 1 tbsp. avocado oil

For the seasoning:

- ½ tsp. garlic powder
- ⅔ tsp. salt
- ½ tsp. ground black pepper

Directions

1. Spiralized zucchini into noodles, place them into a colander, sprinkle with ⅓ tsp. salt, toss until mixed, and set aside until required.
2. Meanwhile, prepare fish and for this, season fillets with the remaining salt and ¾ tsp. Cajun seasoning.
3. Take a medium skillet pan, place it over medium heat, add butter and when it melts, add prepared fillets, switch heat to medium-high level and cook for 3–4 minutes per side until cooked and nicely browned.
4. Transfer fillets to a plate and then reserve the pan for zucchini noodles.
5. Squeeze moisture from the noodles, add them to the skillet pan, add oil, toss until mixed, season with remaining Cajun seasoning, and cook for 2–3 minutes until noodles have turned soft.
6. Sprinkle with garlic powder, remove the pan from heat and distribute noodles between two plates.
7. Top noodles with a fillet and then serve.

Nutrition

- Calories: 350
- Fat: 25 g.
- Protein: 27.1 g.
- Net carb: 2.8 g.

- Fiber: 1.6 g.

24. Garlic Parmesan Mahi-Mahi

Preparation time: 10 minutes
Cooking time: 10 minutes
Servings: 2

Ingredients

- 2 fillets of mahi-mahi
- 1 tsp. minced garlic
- ⅓ tsp. dried thyme
- 1 tbsp. avocado oil
- 1 tbsp. grated parmesan cheese

For the seasoning:

- ⅓ tsp. salt
- ¼ tsp. ground black pepper

Directions

1. Turn on the oven, set it to 425°F, and let it preheat.
2. Meanwhile, take a small bowl, place oil in it, add garlic, thyme, cheese, and oil, and stir until mixed.
3. Season fillets with salt and black pepper, then coat with prepared cheese mixture, place fillets in a baking sheet, and then cook for 7–10 minutes until thoroughly cooked.
4. Serve.

Nutrition

- Calories: 170
- Fat: 7.8 g.
- Net carb: 0.8 g.
- Protein: 22.3 g.
- Fiber: 0 g.

Dinner Recipes

25. Paprika Roasted Radishes With Onions

Preparation time: 20 minutes
Cooking time: 20 minutes
Servings: 4

Ingredients

- 2 large bunches of radishes
- 3 small onion
- 2 tbsp. butter
- 2 tbsp. olive oil
- 1 tsp. fennel seeds
- ½ tsp. smoked paprika
- Sea salt and black pepper

Directions

1. Preheat stove to 350°F. Line a rimmed preparing sheet with material paper.
2. In a blending bowl, consolidate radishes and onion.
3. To the bowl, include spread, olive oil, fennel seeds, paprika, ocean salt, and dark pepper.
4. Remove until radishes and onions are uniformly covered.
5. Pour radishes and onions in a solitary layer onto the material paper.
6. Pour any additional spread and flavoring over the top. Prepare for 20 minutes.

Nutrition

- Calories: 289
- Carbs: 3.2 g.
- Fat: 21.8 g.
- Protein: 12.3 g.

26. Cheesy Roasted Vegetable Spaghetti

Preparation time: 10 minutes
Cooking time: 35 minutes
Servings: 4

Ingredients

- 2 (8 oz.) packs of shirataki spaghetti
- 1 cup chopped mixed bell peppers
- ½ cup grated Parmesan cheese for topping
- 1 lb. asparagus, chopped

- 1 cup broccoli florets
- 1 cup green beans, chopped
- 3 tbsp. olive oil
- 1 small onion, chopped
- 2 garlic cloves, minced
- 1 cup diced tomatoes
- ½ cup chopped basil

Directions

1. Boil 2 cups of water in a pot. Strain the shirataki pasta and rinse well under hot running water. Allow draining and pour the shirataki pasta into the boiling water.
2. Cook for 3 minutes and strain again. Place a dry skillet and stir-fry the shirataki pasta until visibly dry, 1–2 minutes; set aside.
3. Preheat oven to 425°F. In a bowl, add asparagus, broccoli, bell peppers, and green beans and toss with half of the olive oil. Bring the vegetables on a baking sheet and roast for 20 minutes.
4. Heat the remaining olive oil in a skillet and sauté onion and garlic for 3 minutes. Stir in tomatoes and cook for 8 minutes. Mix in shirataki and vegetables.
5. Top with Parmesan cheese and serve.

Nutrition

- Calories: 272
- Fat: 12 g.
- Net carbs: 7 g.
- Protein: 12 g.

27. Garlic 'n Sour Cream Zucchini Bake

Preparation time: 10 minutes
Cooking time: 35 minutes
Servings: 3

Ingredients

- 1 ½ cups zucchini slices
- 5 tbsp. olive oil
- 1 tbsp. minced garlic
- ¼ cup grated Parmesan cheese
- 1 (8 oz.) package of cream cheese, softened
- Salt and pepper to taste

Directions

1. Lightly grease a baking sheet using cooking spray.
2. Place zucchini in a bowl and put in olive oil and garlic.
3. Place zucchini slices in a single layer in a dish.
4. Bake for 35 minutes at 390°F until crispy.
5. In a bowl, whisk well, remaining ingredients.
6. Serve with zucchini.

Nutrition

- Calories: 385
- Carbs: 9.5 g.
- Fat: 32.4 g.
- Protein: 11.9 g.

28. Paprika 'n Cajun Seasoned Onion Rings

Preparation time: 15 minutes
Cooking time: 25 minutes
Servings: 6

Ingredients

- 1 large white onion
- 2 large eggs, beaten
- ½ tsp. Cajun seasoning
- ¾ cup almond flour
- 1 ½ tsp. paprika
- ½ cups coconut oil for frying
- ¼ cup water
- Salt and pepper to taste

Directions

1. Preheat a pot with oil for 8 minutes.
2. Peel the onion cut off the top and slice into circles.

3. In a mixing bowl, combine the water and the eggs. Season with pepper and salt.
4. Soak the onion in the egg mixture.
5. In another bowl, combine the almond flour, paprika powder, Cajun seasoning, salt, and pepper. Dredge the onion in the almond flour mixture.
6. Place in the pot and cook in batches until golden brown, around 8 minutes per batch.

Nutrition

- Calories: 262
- Carbs: 3.9 g.
- Fat: 24.1 g.
- Protein: 2.8 g.

29. Grilled Parmesan Eggplant

Preparation time: 5 minutes
Cooking time: 15 minutes
Servings: 4

Ingredients

- 1 medium-sized eggplant
- 1 (1 lb.) log of fresh mozzarella cheese, cut into sixteen
- 1 small tomato, cut into eight slices
- ½ cup shredded Parmesan cheese
- 1 cup chopped fresh basil or parsley
- ½ tsp. salt
- 1 tbsp. olive oil
- ½ tsp. pepper

Directions

1. Trim ends of the eggplant; cut eggplant crosswise into eight slices. Dust with salt; let stand 5 minutes.
2. Blot eggplant dry with paper towels; brush each side with oil and sprinkle with pepper. Grill, covered, over medium heat 4–6 minutes on each side or until tender. Remove from grill.
3. Top eggplant with mozzarella cheese, tomato, and Parmesan cheese. Grill, covered, 1–2 minutes longer or until cheese begins to melt. Top with basil.

Nutrition

- Calories: 449
- Carbs: 10 g.
- Fat: 31 g.
- Protein: 26 g.

30. Teriyaki Beef Stir-Fry

Preparation time: 10 minutes
Cooking time: 15 minutes
Servings: 6

Ingredients

- 1 ½ tbsp. toasted sesame seed oil
- 1 ½ lb. bottom round steak, cut into bite-sized pieces
- 1 zucchini, sliced
- 1 onion, sliced
- 2 tbsp. coconut aminos
- ½ lime, zested, and juiced
- 2 garlic cloves, grated
- 1 tsp. fresh ginger, minced
- ½ tsp. red pepper flakes, crushed
- 2 tbsp. rice vinegar
- 1 (0.07 oz.) package of stevia

Directions

1. Warm 1 tablespoon of oil in a wok over medium-high heat. Sear the beef for 5–6 minutes until brown around the edges; reserve.
2. Heat the remaining ½ tablespoon of sesame oil and stir fry the zucchini and onion for about 5 minutes.
3. Meanwhile, mix the remaining ingredients to make the sauce.
4. Put the sauce into the wok; return the reserved beef to the wok. Cook approximately 3 minutes over medium-high heat until thoroughly heated. Serve immediately.

Nutrition

- Calories: 207
- Fat: 11 g.
- Carbs: 1.1 g.
- Protein: 24.2 g.
- Fiber: 0.1 g.

31. Grilled Beef Short Loin

Preparation time: 5 minutes
Cooking time: 25 minutes
Servings: 2

Ingredients

- 1 ½ lb. beef short loin
- 2 thyme sprigs, chopped
- 1 rosemary sprig, chopped
- 1 tsp. garlic powder
- Sea salt, to taste
- Ground black pepper, to taste

Directions

1. Bring all of the above ingredients in a re-sealable zipper bag. Shake until the beef short loin is well coated on all sides.
2. Cook on a preheated grill for 15–20 minutes, flipping once or twice during the cooking time.
3. Let it stand for 5 minutes before slicing and serving. Bon appétit!

Nutrition

- Calories: 313
- Carbs: 0.1 g.
- Fat: 11.6 g.
- Fiber: 0.1 g.
- Protein: 52 g.

32. Intermittent Roasted Bone Marrow

Preparation time: 5 minutes
Cooking time: 20 minutes
Servings: 2

Ingredients

- 4 bone marrow halves
- Sea salt to taste
- Freshly ground black pepper to taste

Directions

1. Preheat the stove to 350°F.
2. Spot the bones marrow side-up onto a profound preparing plate.
3. Spot in the broiler for 20–25 minutes until brilliant and firm, and the vast majority of the overabundance fat has rendered off.
4. Season the marrow with ocean salt chips and naturally ground dark pepper.
5. Serve without anyone else as a starter or scoop out the marrow and spread on flame-broiled steak.

Nutrition

- Calories: 440
- Carbs: 1.4 g.
- Fat: 48 g.
- Protein: 4 g.

33. Intermittent Spicy Beef Avocado Cups

Preparation time: 5 minutes
Cooking time: 15 minutes
Servings: 2

Ingredients

- 1 beefsteak, chopped into small cubes
- 2 chili peppers
- ½ medium onion
- 2 tbsp. avocado oil
- 2 tbsp. gluten-free tamari sauce or coconut amino
- 1 large ripe avocado

Directions

1. Add the avocado oil to a skillet on high fire and cook the steak three-D shapes till accomplished simply as you will prefer.

2. Add peppers and onions to the skillet and prepare dinner until mellowed.
3. Utilize regularly avocado oil if required. Return the steak blocks to the skillet and season with tamari sauce.
4. Spoon the beef combination over the avocado components and serve.

Nutrition

- Calories: 570
- Fat: 50 g.
- Carbs: 6.3 g.
- Protein: 19 g.

34. Intermittent Rosemary Roast Beef and White Radishes

Preparation time: 10 minutes
Cooking time: 60 minutes
Servings: 8

Ingredients

- 3 lb. boneless beef roast
- 2 white daikon radishes
- 3 tbsp. rosemary
- 2 tbsp. salt, to taste
- 2 tbsp. olive oil

Directions

1. Preheat oven to 400°F.
2. Spread olive oil, rosemary, and salt over the cheeseburger.
3. Place the stripped and severed radishes at the base of a warming dish.
4. Place the burger over the radishes and warmth for an hour.
5. Wrap the burger by utilizing foil and permit unwinding for 20 minutes sooner than serving.

Nutrition

- Calories: 492
- Carbs: 4.1 g.
- Fat: 39 g.
- Protein: 29 g.

35. Intermittent Beef Liver With Asian Dip

Preparation time: 10 minutes
Cooking time: 15 minutes
Servings: 10

Ingredients

- 1 lb. beef liver, whole
- ¼ cup tamari sauce
- 2 cloves garlic
- 1 tsp. fresh ginger
- 1 tsp. sesame oil

Directions

1. Spot the meat liver into a pot secured with water and heat to the point of boiling. Bubble for 2–3 minutes and afterward pour the water with the filth out. Top off with new water and bubble for 10 minutes.
2. In the interim, make the plunge by combining all the plunge ingredients.
3. Let the hamburger liver cool, at that point, cut it daintily and appreciate with the plunge.

Nutrition

- Calories: 66
- Carbs: 2 g.
- Fat: 2 g.
- Protein: 9 g.

36. Chinese Bok Choy and Turkey Soup

Preparation time: 15 minutes
Cooking time: 40 minutes
Servings: 8

Ingredients

- ½ lb. baby bok choy, sliced into quarters lengthwise
- 2 lb. turkey carcass
- 1 tbsp. olive oil
- ½ cup leeks, chopped

- 1 celery rib, chopped
- 2 carrots, sliced
- 6 cups turkey stock
- Himalayan salt and black pepper, to taste

Directions

1. In a heavy-bottomed pot, heat the olive oil until sizzling. Once hot, sauté the celery, carrots, leek, and Bok choy for about 6 minutes.
2. Add the salt, pepper, turkey, and stock; bring to a boil.
3. Turn the heat to simmer. Continue to cook, partially covered, for about 35 minutes.

Nutrition

- Calories: 211
- Carbs: 3.1 g.
- Fat: 11.8 g.
- Fiber: 0.9 g.
- Protein: 23.7 g.

Appetizers and Snacks

37. Appealing Broccoli Mash

Preparation time: 15 minutes
Cooking time: 5 minutes
Servings: 6

Ingredients

- 16 oz. broccoli florets
- 1 cup water
- 1 tsp. fresh lemon juice
- 1 tsp. butter, softened
- 1 tsp. garlic, minced
- Salt and freshly ground black pepper, to taste

Directions

1. In a medium pan, add the broccoli and water over medium heat and cook for about 5 minutes.
2. Drain the broccoli well and transfer into a large bowl
3. In the bowl of broccoli, add the lemon juice, butter, and garlic, and with an immersion blender blend until smooth.
4. Season with salt and black pepper and serve.

Nutrition

- Calories: 32
- Carbohydrates: 5.1 g.
- Fat: 0.9 g.
- Fiber: 2 g.
- Protein: 2 g.
- Sodium: 160 mg.
- Sugar: 1.3 g.

38. Zesty Brussels Sprout

Preparation time: 15 minutes
Cooking time: 15 minutes
Servings: 2

Ingredients

- ½ lb. fresh Brussels sprouts, trimmed and halved
- 2 tbsp. olive oil
- 2 small garlic cloves, minced
- ½ tsp. red pepper flakes, crushed
- Salt and freshly ground black pepper, to taste
- 1 tbsp. fresh lemon juice
- 1 tsp. fresh lemon zest, grated finely

Directions

1. Arrange a steamer basket over a large pan of boiling water.
2. Place the asparagus into the steamer basket and steam, covered for about 6–8 minutes.
3. Remove from the heat and drain the asparagus well.
4. In a large skillet, heat the oil over medium heat and sauté the garlic and red pepper flakes for about 1 minute. Stir in the Brussels sprouts, salt, and black pepper, and sauté for about 4–5 minutes. Stir in the lemon juice and sauté for about 1 minute more.
5. Remove from the heat and serve hot with the garnishing of the lemon zest.

Nutrition

- Calories: 116
- Carbohydrates: 11 g.
- Fat: 7.5 g.
- Fiber: 4.4 g.
- Protein: 4.1 g.
- Sodium: 102 mg.
- Sugar: 2.5 g.

39. Simplest Yellow Squash

Preparation time: 10 minutes
Cooking time: 12 minutes
Servings: 4

Ingredients

- 2 tbsp. olive oil
- 1 lb. yellow squash, cut into thin slices
- 1 small yellow onion, cut into thin rings
- 1 garlic clove, minced
- 3 tsp. water
- Salt and freshly ground white pepper, to taste

Directions

1. In a large skillet, heat the oil over medium-high heat and stir fry the squash, onion, and garlic for about 3–4 minutes.
2. Add water, salt, and black pepper and stir to combine.
3. Reduce heat to low and simmer for about 6–8 minutes.
4. Serve hot.

Nutrition

- Calories: 86
- Carbohydrates: 5.7 g.
- Fat: 7.2 g.
- Fiber: 1.7 g.
- Protein: 1.6 g.
- Sodium: 51 mg.
- Sugar: 2.7 g.

40. Pumpkin and Cauliflower Rice

Preparation time: 5 minutes
Cooking time: 10 minutes
Servings: 4

Ingredients

- 2 oz. olive oil
- 1 yellow onion, chopped
- 2 garlic cloves, minced
- 12 oz. cauliflower rice
- 4 cups chicken stock
- 6 oz. pumpkin puree
- ½ tsp. nutmeg, ground
- 1 tsp. thyme chopped
- ½ tsp. ginger, grated
- ½ tsp. cinnamon powder
- ½ tsp. allspice
- 4 oz. coconut cream

Directions

1. Set your instant pot on sauté mode, add the oil, heat it up, and add garlic and onion, stir and sauté for 3 minutes.
2. Add cauliflower rice, stock, pumpkin puree, thyme, nutmeg, cinnamon, ginger, and allspice, stir, cover, and cook on high for 12 minutes.
3. Add coconut cream, stir, divide among plates and serve as a side dish.
4. Enjoy!

Nutrition

- Calories: 152
- Carbs: 5 g.
- Fat: 2 g.
- Fiber: 3 g.
- Protein: 6 g.

41. Special Collard Greens

Preparation time: 10 minutes
Cooking time: 5 minutes
Servings: 4

Ingredients

- 1 tbsp. olive oil
- 16 oz. collard greens
- 1 cup yellow onion, chopped
- 2 garlic cloves, minced

- A pinch of sea salt and black pepper
- 14 oz. veggie stock
- 1 bay leaf
- 3 tbsp. balsamic vinegar

Directions

1. Set your instant pot on sauté mode, add the oil, heat it up, and add onion, stir and sauté for 3 minutes.
2. Add collard greens, stir and sauté for 2 minutes more.
3. Add garlic, salt, pepper, stock, and bay leaf, stir, cover and cook on high for 5 minutes.
4. Add vinegar, toss, divide among plates, and serve.
5. Enjoy!

Nutrition

- Calories: 130
- Carbs: 3 g.
- Fat: 1 g.
- Fiber: 2 g.
- Protein: 5 g.

42. Instant Zucchini With Green Peppercorn Sauce

Preparation time: 2 minutes
Cooking time: 10 minutes
Servings: 4

Ingredients

- 1 cup water
- 2 zucchini, sliced
- Sea salt, to taste

For the green peppercorn sauce:

- 2 tbsp. butter
- ½ cup green onions, minced
- 2 tbsp. cognac
- 1 ½ cups chicken broth
- 1 cup whipping cream
- 1 ½ tbsp. green peppercorns in brine, drained and crushed slightly

Directions

1. Add water and a steamer basket to the Instant Pot. Arrange your zucchini on the steamer basket.
2. Secure the lid. Choose "Manual" mode and low pressure; cook for 3 minutes. Once cooking is complete, use a quick pressure release; carefully remove the lid.
3. Season zucchini with salt and set aside.
4. Wipe down the Instant Pot with a damp cloth. Press the "Sauté" button to heat up your Instant Pot.
5. Melt the butter and then, sauté green onions until tender. Add cognac and cook for 2 minutes longer. Then, pour in chicken broth and let it boil for another 4 minutes.
6. Lastly, stir in the cream and peppercorns. Continue to simmer until the sauce is thickened and thoroughly warmed.
7. Serve your zucchini with the sauce on the side. Bon appétit!

Nutrition

- Calories: 251
- Fat: 15.3 g.
- Total carbs: 3.2 g.
- Protein: 20.2 g.
- Sugars: 1.5 g.

43. Lazy Sunday Mushroom Ragout

Preparation time: 2 minutes
Cooking time: 10 minutes
Servings: 4

Ingredients

- 3 tbsp. butter, at room temperature
- ½ cup white onions, peeled and sliced
- 1 cup chicken sausage, casing removed, sliced
- 1 lb. Chanterelle mushrooms, sliced
- 2 stalks spring garlic, diced
- Kosher salt and ground black pepper, to taste

- ½ tsp. red pepper flakes
- 2 tbsp. tomato paste
- ½ cup good Pinot Noir
- 1 cup chicken stock
- ½ cup double cream
- 2 tbsp. fresh chives, chopped

Directions

1. Press the "Sauté" button to heat up your Instant Pot. Once hot, melt the butter and sauté the onions until tender and translucent.
2. Add the sausage and mushrooms; continue to sauté until the sausage is no longer pink and the mushrooms are fragrant.
3. Then, stir in garlic and cook it for 30–40 seconds more or until aromatic. Now, add the salt, black pepper, red pepper, tomato paste, Pinot Noir, and chicken stock.
4. Secure the lid. Choose "Manual" mode and High pressure; cook for 5 minutes. Once cooking is complete, use a quick pressure release; carefully remove the lid.
5. After that, add the double cream and press the "Sauté" button. Continue to simmer until everything is heated through and slightly thickened.
6. Lastly, divide your stew among individual bowls; top with fresh chopped chives and serve warm.

Nutrition

- Calories: 279
- Fat: 22.3 g.
- Total carbs: 6.3 g.
- Protein: 8.7 g.
- Sugars: 3.2 g.

44. Rolls of Sausage Pizzas

Preparation time: 10 minutes
Cooking time: 30 minutes
Servings: 6

Ingredients

- ¼ cup. pizza sauce
- 2 cup. shredded mozzarella cheese
- ½ cup. cooked sausage
- Salt
- 1 tsp. pizza seasoning
- 2 tbsp. chopped onion
- Black pepper
- ¼ cup. chopped red and green bell peppers
- 1 cup chopped tomato

Directions

1. Line a baking sheet. Grease it slightly. Over the sheet, spread mozzarella cheese and top with sprinkles of pizza seasoning. Set in an oven preheated to 400°F and bake until done for 20 minutes.
2. Remove the pizza crust from the oven. Spread it with tomatoes, sausage, bell peppers, and onion. Top with tomato sauce drizzling.
3. Put it back in the oven and bake for another 10 minutes. Remove the pizza from the oven and allow it to cool. Slice into 6 equal parts and roll. Enjoy your lunch.

Nutrition

- Calories: 117
- Carbs: 2 g.
- Fat: 7 g.
- Fiber: 1 g.
- Protein: 11 g.

45. Stuffed Sausage With Bacon Wrappings

Preparation time: 10 minutes
Cooking time: 15 minutes
Servings: 4

Ingredients

- Onion powder
- Bacon strips
- Salt
- Garlic powder

- Black pepper
- Sausages
- ½ tsp. sweet paprika
- 16 pepper jack cheese slices

Directions

1. Ensure you have a medium-high source of heat. Set a grill on it. Add sausages to cook until done on all sides and set on a plate to cool.
2. Slice a pocket opening in the sausages. Each to be stuffed with 2 slices of pepper jack cheese. Apply a seasoning of onion, pepper, garlic powder, paprika, and salt.
3. Each stuffed sausage should be wrapped in a bacon strip and grip using a toothpick. Set them on the baking sheet and transfer them to the oven to bake at 400°F for almost 15 minutes.
4. Serve immediately and enjoy.

Nutrition

- Calories: 500
- Carbs: 4 g.
- Fat: 37 g.
- Fiber: 12 g.
- Protein: 40 g.

46. Coated Avocado Tacos

Preparation time: 10 minutes
Cooking time: 20 minutes
Servings: 12

Ingredients

- 1 avocado
- 12 tortillas and toppings
- ½ cup panko breadcrumbs
- 1 egg
- Salt

Directions

1. Scoop out the meat from each avocado shell and slice them into wedges.
2. Beat the egg in a shallow bowl and put the breadcrumbs in another bowl.
3. Dip the avocado wedges in the beaten egg and coat them with breadcrumbs. Sprinkle them with a bit of salt. Arrange them in the cooking basket in a single layer.
4. Cook for 15 minutes at 392°F. Shake the basket halfway through the cooking process.
5. Put the cooked avocado wedges in tortillas and add your preferred toppings.

Nutrition

- Calories: 179
- Fat: 6.07 g.
- Carbs: 26.29 g.
- Protein: 4.94 g.

47. Crispy Potato Skins

Preparation time: 5 minutes
Cooking time: 55 minutes
Servings: 2

Ingredients

- 2 Yukon Gold potatoes
- ¼ tsp. sea salt
- ½ tsp. olive oil
- 2 minced green onions
- 4 bacon strips
- ¼ cup shredded cheddar cheese
- ⅓ cup sour cream

Directions

1. Rinse and scrub the potatoes until clean. Rub with oil and sprinkle with salt. Put them in the cooking basket. Cook for 35 minutes at 400°F. Transfer the cooked potatoes to a platter.
2. Put the bacon strip in the cooking basket. Cook for 5 minutes at 400°F.
3. Move to a plate and leave to cool. Crumble into bits.
4. Slice the potatoes in half.
5. Scoop out most of the meat.

6. Arrange the potato skins with the skin facing side up in the cooking basket. Spray them with oil.
7. Cook for 3 minutes at 400°F. Flip the potato skins.
8. Fill each piece with cheese and crumbled bacon. Continue cooking for 2 more minutes.
9. Transfer to a platter. Add a little portion of sour cream on top. Sprinkle with minced onion and serve while warm.

Nutrition

- Calories: 483
- Fat: 8.73 g.
- Carbs: 92.8 g.
- Protein: 12.52 g.

Salads and Soups

48. Coconut, Green Beans, and Shrimp Curry Soup

Preparation time: 10 minutes
Cooking time: 15 minutes
Servings: 4

Ingredients

- 2 tbsp. ghee
- 1 lb. jumbo shrimp, peeled and deveined
- 2 tsp. ginger-garlic puree
- 2 tbsp. red curry paste
- 6 oz. coconut milk
- Salt and chili pepper to taste
- 1 bunch green beans, halved

Directions

1. Melt ghee in a medium saucepan over medium heat.
2. Add the shrimp, season with salt and black pepper, and cook until they are opaque, 2–3 minutes.
3. Remove shrimp to a plate.
4. Add the ginger-garlic puree and red curry paste to the ghee and sauté for 2 minutes until fragrant.
5. Stir in the coconut milk; add the shrimp, salt, chili pepper, and green beans.
6. Cook for 4 minutes.
7. Reduce the heat to a simmer and cook an additional 3 minutes, occasionally stirring.
8. Adjust taste with salt, fetch soup into serving bowls, and serve with cauliflower rice.

Nutrition

- Calories: 375
- Fat: 35.4 g.
- Net carbs: 2 g.
- Protein: 9 g.

49. Salsa Verde Chicken Soup

Preparation time: 5 minutes
Cooking time: 10 minutes
Servings: 4

Ingredients

- ½ cup Salsa Verde
- 2 cups cooked and shredded chicken
- 2 cups chicken broth
- 1 cup shredded cheddar cheese
- 4 oz. cream cheese
- ½ tsp. chili powder
- ½ tsp. ground cumin
- ½ tsp. fresh cilantro, chopped
- Salt and black pepper, to taste

Directions

1. Combine the cream cheese, Salsa Verde, and broth, in a food processor; pulse until smooth. Transfer the mixture to a pot and place over medium heat.
2. Cook until hot, but do not bring to a boil. Add chicken, chili powder, and cumin and cook for about 3–5 minutes, or until it is heated through.
3. Stir in cheddar cheese and season with salt and pepper to taste. If it is very thick, add a few tbsp. water and boil for 1–3 more

minutes. Serve hot in bowls sprinkled with fresh cilantro.

Nutrition

- Calories: 346
- Fat: 23 g.
- Net carbs: 3 g.
- Protein: 25 g.

50. Creamy Squash Soup

Preparation time: 15 minutes
Cooking time: 30 minutes
Servings: 10

Ingredients

- 10 cups butternut squash, cubed
- 1 tbsp. olive oil
- 1 onion, chopped
- 4 cloves garlic, minced
- 1 ½ tsp. salt
- ½ tsp. black pepper
- 5 cups vegetable stock
- 1 cup heavy cream

Directions

1. Heat the oil in a heavy skillet over medium-high heat. Add onion, garlic, salt, pepper, and sauté, stirring, until the onion is translucent.
2. Add squash and stock to a large pot. Transfer vegetables to the pot.
3. Bring to a low simmer and cook until the squash is tender, for about 20–30 minutes. Add water if necessary, during cooking.
4. Add the cream, stirring to combine. If you have an immersion blender, use it to puree the soup in the pot. If not, transfer the soup to a blender or food processor and blend it to a smooth puree.
5. Serve warm.

Nutrition

- Calories: 62
- Carbohydrates: 9 g.
- Fat: 22 g.
- Protein: 3 g.

51. Cauliflower Cheese Soup

Preparation time: 10 minutes
Cooking time: 30 minutes
Servings: 4

Ingredients

- 1 head cauliflower, chopped
- ½ onion, chopped
- 2 tbsp. olive oil
- 3 cups chicken stock
- 1 tsp. garlic powder
- 1 tsp. kosher salt
- 4 oz. cream cheese, cubed
- 1 cup cheddar cheese, grated
- ½ cup milk

Directions

1. Heat the oil in a heavy stockpot over medium-high heat. Add onion and cook until softened, about 3 minutes. Add cauliflower, stock, salt, and garlic powder.
2. Bring to a low simmer and cook until the cauliflower is tender, for about 20 minutes. Add water if necessary, during cooking.
3. Transfer cauliflower to a blender or food processor and blend to a smooth puree.
4. Return pureed cauliflower to the pot and add the cream cheese and cheddar cheese, stirring as the mixture heats over medium-low heat.
5. When the cheese has melted, add the milk and heat thoroughly.

Nutrition

- Calories: 51
- Carbohydrates: 17 g.
- Protein: 5 g.
- Total fat: 8 g.

52. Chilled Avocado Tomato Soup

Preparation time: 7 minutes
Cooking time: 20 minutes

Servings: 1–2

Ingredients

- 2 small avocados
- 2 large tomatoes
- 1 stalk of celery
- 1 small onion
- 1 clove of garlic
- Juice of 1 fresh lemon
- 1 cup of water (best: alkaline water)
- A handful of fresh lavage
- Parsley and sea salt to taste

Directions

1. Scoop the avocados and cut all veggies into little pieces.
2. Spot all the ingredients in a blender and blend until smooth.
3. Serve chilled and appreciate this nutritious and sound-soluble soup formula!

Nutrition

- Calories: 68
- Carbohydrates: 15 g.
- Fat: 2 g.
- Protein: 0.8 g.

53. Baked "Potato" Salad

Preparation time: 6 minutes
Cooking time: 15 minutes
Servings: 8

Ingredients

- 2 lb. cauliflower, separated into small florets
- 6–8 slices bacon, chopped and fried crisp
- 6 boiled eggs, cooled, peeled, and chopped
- 1 cup sharp cheddar cheese, grated
- ½ cup green onion, sliced
- 1 cup reduced-fat mayonnaise
- 2 tsp. yellow mustard
- 1 ½ tsp. onion powder, divided
- Salt and fresh-ground black pepper to taste

Directions

1. Place cauliflower in a vegetable steamer, or a pot with a steamer insert, and steam for 5–6 minutes. Drain the cauliflower and set it aside.
2. In a small bowl, whisk together mayonnaise, mustard, 1 tsp. onion powder, salt, and pepper.
3. Pat cauliflower dry with paper towels and place in a large mixing bowl.
4. Add eggs, salt, pepper, remaining ½ tsp. onion powder, then dressing.
5. Mix gently to combine ingredients together.
6. Fold in the bacon, cheese, and green onion. Serve warm or cover and chill before serving.

Nutrition

- Calories: 247
- Fat: 17 g.
- Protein: 17 g.

54. Caprese Salad

Preparation time: 6 minutes
Cooking time: 15 minutes
Servings: 4

Ingredients

- 3 medium tomatoes, cut into 8 slices
- 2 (1 oz.) slices of mozzarella cheese, cut into strips
- ¼ cup fresh basil, sliced thin
- 2 tsp. extra-virgin olive oil
- ⅛ tsp. salt
- Pinch black pepper

Directions

1. Place tomatoes and cheese on serving plates.
2. Sprinkle with salt and pepper.
3. Drizzle oil over and top with basil.
4. Serve.

Nutrition

- Calories: 77
- Fat: 5 g.
- Protein: 5 g.

55. Broccoli Salad

Preparation time: 10 minutes
Cooking time: none
Servings: 6

Ingredients

- 1 medium head broccoli, raw, florets only
- ½ cup red onion, chopped
- 12 oz. turkey bacon, chopped, fried until crisp
- ½ cup cherry tomatoes, halved
- ¼ cup sunflower kernels
- ¾ cup raisins
- ¾ cup mayonnaise
- 2 tbsp. white vinegar

Directions

1. In a salad bowl combine the broccoli, tomatoes, and onion.
2. Mix mayo with vinegar and sprinkle over the broccoli.
3. Add the sunflower kernels, raisins, and bacon, and toss well.

Nutrition

- Calories: 220
- Carbohydrates: 17.3 g.
- Protein: 11 g.

56. Asian Cucumber Salad

Preparation time: 10 minutes
Cooking time: 0 minute
Servings: 6

Ingredients

- 1 lb. cucumbers, sliced
- 2 scallions, sliced
- 2 tbsp. sliced pickled ginger, chopped
- ¼ cup cilantro
- ½ red jalapeño, chopped
- 3 tbsp. rice wine vinegar
- 1 tbsp. sesame oil
- 1 tbsp. sesame seeds

Directions

1. In a salad bowl combine all ingredients and toss together.

Nutrition

- Calories: 52
- Carbohydrates: 5.7 g.
- Protein: 1 g.

57. Chicken Salad in Cucumber Cups

Preparation time: 5 minutes
Cooking time: 15 minutes
Servings: 4

Ingredients

- ½ chicken breast, skinless, boiled, and shredded
- 2 long cucumbers, cut into 8 thick rounds each, scooped out
- 1 tsp. ginger, minced
- 1 tsp. lime zest, grated
- 4 tsp. olive oil
- 1 tsp. sesame oil
- 1 tsp. lime juice
- Salt and pepper to taste

Directions

1. In a bowl combine lime zest, juice, olive and sesame oils, ginger, and season with salt.
2. Toss the chicken with the dressing and fill the cucumber cups with the salad.

Nutrition

- Calories: 116 g.
- Carbohydrates: 4 g.
- Protein: 12 g.

58. Sunflower Seeds and Arugula Garden Salad

Preparation time: 5 minutes
Cooking time: 10 minutes

Servings: 6

Ingredients

- ¼ tsp. black pepper
- ¼ tsp. salt
- 1 tsp. fresh thyme, chopped
- 2 tbsp. sunflower seeds, toasted
- 2 cups red grapes, halved
- 7 cups baby arugula, loosely packed
- 1 tbsp. coconut oil
- 2 tsp. honey
- 3 tbsp. red wine vinegar
- ½ tsp. stone-ground mustard

Directions

1. In a small bowl, whisk together mustard, honey, and vinegar. Slowly pour oil as you whisk.
2. In a large salad bowl, mix thyme, seeds, grapes, and arugula.
3. Drizzle with dressing and serve.

Nutrition

- Calories: 86.7
- Fat: 3.1 g.
- Protein: 1.6 g.

59. Supreme Caesar Salad

Preparation time: 5 minutes
Cooking time: 10 minutes
Servings: 4

Ingredients

- ¼ cup olive oil
- ¾ cup mayonnaise
- 1 head Romaine lettuce, torn into bite-sized pieces
- 1 tbsp. lemon juice
- 1 tsp. Dijon mustard
- 1 tsp. Worcestershire sauce
- 3 cloves garlic, peeled and minced
- 3 cloves garlic, peeled and quartered
- 4 cups day-old bread, cubed
- 5 anchovy filets, minced
- 6 tbsp. grated parmesan cheese, divided
- Ground black pepper to taste
- Salt to taste

Directions

1. In a small bowl, whisk well lemon juice, mustard, Worcestershire sauce, 2 tbsp. parmesan cheese, anchovies, mayonnaise, and minced garlic. Season with pepper and salt to taste. Set aside in the ref.
2. On medium fire, place a large nonstick saucepan and heat oil.
3. Sauté quartered garlic until browned around a minute or two. Remove and discard.
4. Add bread cubes in the same pan, sauté until lightly browned. Season with pepper and salt. Transfer to a plate.
5. In a large bowl, place lettuce and pour in the dressing. Toss well to coat. Top with remaining parmesan cheese.
6. Garnish with bread cubes, serve, and enjoy.

Nutrition

- Calories: 443.3 g.
- Fat: 32.1 g.
- Protein: 11.6 g.

Meat Recipes

60. Beef With Cabbage Noodles

Preparation time: 5 minutes
Cooking time: 18 minutes
Servings: 2

Ingredients

- 4 oz. ground beef
- 1 cup chopped cabbage
- 4 oz. tomato sauce
- ½ tsp. minced garlic
- ½ cup of water
- ½ tbsp. coconut oil
- ½ tsp. salt
- ¼ tsp. Italian seasoning
- ⅛ tsp. dried basil

Directions

1. Take a skillet pan, place it over medium heat, add oil and when hot, add beef and cook for 5 minutes until nicely browned.
2. Meanwhile, prepare the cabbage and for it, slice the cabbage into thin shred.
3. When the beef has cooked, add garlic, season with salt, basil, and Italian seasoning, stir well and continue cooking for 3 minutes until beef has thoroughly cooked.
4. Pour in tomato sauce and water, stir well and bring the mixture to boil.
5. Then reduce heat to medium-low level, add cabbage, stir well until well mixed and simmer for 3–5 minutes until cabbage is softened, covering the pan.
6. Uncover the pan and continue simmering the beef until most of the cooking liquid has evaporated.
7. Serve.

Nutrition

- Calories: 188.5
- Fat: 12.5 g.
- Protein: 15.5 g.
- Net carb: 2.5 g.
- Fiber: 1 g.

61. **Roast Beef and Mozzarella Plate**

Preparation time: 5 minutes
Cooking time: 0 minutes
Servings: 2

Ingredients

- 4 slices of roast beef
- ½ oz. chopped lettuce
- 1 avocado, pitted
- 2 oz. mozzarella cheese, cubed
- ½ cup mayonnaise
- ¼ tsp. salt
- ⅛ tsp. ground black pepper
- 2 tbsp. avocado oil

Directions

1. Scoop out flesh from avocado and divide it evenly between two plates.
2. Add slices of roast beef, lettuce, and cheese, and then sprinkle with salt and black pepper.
3. Serve with avocado oil and mayonnaise.

Nutrition

- Calories: 267.7
- Fat: 24.5 g.
- Fiber: 2 g.
- Net carb: 1.5 g.
- Protein: 9.5 g.

62. **Garlic Herb Beef Roast**

Preparation time: 5 minutes
Cooking time: 10 minutes
Servings: 2

Ingredients

- 6 slices of beef roast
- ½ tsp. garlic powder
- ⅓ tsp. dried thyme
- ¼ tsp. dried rosemary
- 2 tbsp. butter, unsalted
- ⅓ tsp. salt
- ¼ tsp. ground black pepper

Directions

1. Prepare the spice mix and for this, take a small bowl, place garlic powder, thyme, rosemary, salt, and black pepper and then stir until mixed.
2. Sprinkle spice mix on the beef roast.
3. Take a medium skillet pan, place it over medium heat, add butter and when it melts, add beef roast and then cook for 5–8 minutes until golden brown and cooked.
4. Serve.

Nutrition

- Calories: 140
- Fat: 12.7 g.
- Fiber: 0.2 g.
- Net carb: 0.1 g.
- Protein: 5.5 g.

63. Grilled Pork Patties

Preparation time: 10 minutes
Cooking time: 7–8 minutes
Servings: 6

Ingredients

- 1 ½ lb. ground pork
- ½ lb. ground turkey
- 1 serrano pepper, deseeded and minced
- 2 garlic cloves, finely minced
- ½ cup onion, finely minced
- 1 cup Romano cheese, grated
- ½ cup Asiago cheese, shredded
- 1 tsp. mustard seeds
- ½ tsp. dried marjoram
- ½ tsp. dried basil
- 1 tsp. paprika
- Sea salt, to taste
- Ground black pepper, to taste

Directions

1. Begin by preheating a gas grill to high.
2. Mix all of the above ingredients until everything is well incorporated. Form the mixture into 6 patties with oiled hands.
3. Place on the preheated grill and cook for 7–8 minutes on each side until slightly charred. Bon appétit!

Nutrition

- Calories: 515
- Fat: 35.4 g.
- Carbs: 2.6 g.
- Protein: 44.3 g.
- Fiber: 0.2 g.

64. Pork Fillets With Mustard Sauce

Preparation time: 10 minutes
Cooking time: 20 minutes
Servings: 4

Ingredients

- 4 tbsp. butter, melted
- 1 lb. pork fillets
- 2 scallions, chopped
- 2 cloves garlic, minced
- ½ cup dry white wine
- Sea salt, to taste
- Freshly cracked black pepper, to taste
- 1 tsp. cayenne pepper
- 1 tsp. dried basil
- 2 tbsp. whole-grain Dijon mustard
- 2 tbsp. chicken stock

Directions

1. Melt the butter in a frying pan at a moderate flame. Now, brown the pork fillets for about 3 minutes per side; reserve.
2. Then, in the pan drippings, continue to cook the scallions and garlic for a minute or so. Add in a splash of wine to scrape up the browned bits that stick to the pan's bottom.
3. Return the pork to the frying pan. Add in the remaining ingredients, partially cover, and cook for an additional 13 minutes.
4. Spoon the sauce over the pork fillets and serve warm. Bon appétit!

Nutrition

- Calories: 343
- Carbs: 5.4 g.
- Fat: 17.5 g.
- Fiber: 1 g.
- Protein: 40 g.

65. Sunday Ground Pork Bake

Preparation time: 9 minutes

Cooking time: 21 minutes
Servings: 4

Ingredients

- 1 tbsp. butter
- 2 lb. ground pork
- 1 bell pepper, deseeded and chopped
- 1 serrano pepper, deseeded and chopped
- 1 leek, chopped
- 2 garlic cloves, minced
- ½ cup chicken broth
- 2 eggs, beaten
- 1 tsp. paprika
- Sea salt, to taste
- Ground black pepper, to taste
- ½ cup cream cheese
- 1 cup heavy whipped cream

Directions

1. Melt the butter in a frying pan at moderate heat. Now, cook the ground pork until no longer pink.
2. Add in the peppers, leek, and garlic and continue to cook approximately 7 minutes or until tender and aromatic.
3. Pour the chicken broth and continue to cook for a further 6 minutes. Scoop the mixture into a lightly greased baking pan.
4. In a mixing bowl, whisk the egg, paprika, salt, black pepper, cream cheese, and heavy whipped cream. Pour the mixture into the prepared baking pan.
5. Bake in the preheated oven at 330°F for about 8 minutes until golden brown on the top. Bon appétit!

Nutrition

- Calories: 620
- Carbs: 5.7 g.
- Fat: 50 g.
- Fiber: 0.7 g.
- Protein: 33.9 g.

66. Pork Cutlets in Chili Tangy Sauce

Preparation time: 10 minutes
Cooking time: 5 minutes
Servings: 3

Ingredients

- 1 lb. pork cutlets
- Sea salt, to taste
- Ground black pepper, to taste
- ½ tsp. thyme
- ½ tsp. rosemary
- 1 tsp. basil
- 1 tbsp. lard, room temperature

For the sauce:

- 2 tbsp. sherry
- ¼ cup sour cream
- ¼ cup beef bone broth
- 1 tsp. mustard
- ½ tsp. turmeric powder
- ½ tsp. chili powder

Directions

1. Season the pork cutlets using salt, pepper, thyme, rosemary, and basil.
2. Melt the lard in a pan on medium-high heat; now, sear pork cutlets for 3 minutes; flip and cook for 3 minutes on the other side. Reserve.
3. Deglaze your pan with sherry, add the remaining ingredients and cook on medium-low heat until the sauce has thickened slightly.
4. Put the reserved pork and let it simmer for a couple of minutes or until everything is heated through. Scoop the sauce over pork cutlets and serve.

Nutrition

- Calories: 288
- Fat: 17.3 g.
- Carbs: 1.1 g.
- Fiber: 0 g.
- Protein: 29.9 g.

67. Pork Medallions With Aromatic Herb Butter

Preparation time: 10 minutes
Cooking time: 10 minutes
Servings: 6

Ingredients

- 2 tbsp. olive oil
- 6 pork medallions
- 1 tsp. mustard powder
- 1 tsp. paprika
- Sea salt, to taste
- Freshly ground black pepper, to taste
- ⅔ cup butter, at room temperature
- 2 cloves garlic, smashed
- ½ tsp. dried thyme, crushed
- 1 tsp. dried rosemary, crushed
- 1 tbsp. lemon juice

Directions

1. In a frying pan, warm the oil to medium-high heat.
2. Cook the pork medallions for 4–5 minutes per side or until they achieve the reddish-brown exterior.
3. Now, season the pork medallions with mustard powder, paprika, salt, and black pepper.
4. Mix the remaining ingredients in a bowl.
5. Serve the pork medallions with well-chilled herb butter.
6. Enjoy!

Nutrition

- Calories: 451
- Fat: 31.7 g.
- Carbs: 0.8 g.
- Protein: 39.5 g.
- Fiber: 0.2 g.

68. Grilled Back Ribs

Preparation time: 10 minutes
Cooking time: 20 minutes
Servings: 4

Ingredients

- 2 lb. back ribs
- 2 tbsp. coconut aminos
- 1 tsp. garlic powder
- 1 tsp. shallot powder
- 1 tbsp. monk fruit powder
- Sea salt, to taste
- Ground black pepper, to taste
- 2 tbsp. dry red wine
- ½ cup beef bone broth
- 2 tbsp. olive oil

Directions

1. Bring all of the above ingredients in a ceramic dish.
2. Cover and let it marinate in your refrigerator overnight; reserve the marinade.
3. Grill the back ribs over medium-high heat for about 5 minutes per side, basting them with the reserved marinade. An instant thermometer should read 145°F.
4. Serve with mashed cauliflower if desired.
5. Enjoy!

Nutrition

- Calories: 570
- Carbs: 2.1 g.
- Fat: 42.4 g.
- Fiber: 0.3 g.
- Protein: 45 g.

69. Coffee Barbecue Pork Belly

Preparation time: 15 minutes
Cooking time: 60 minutes
Servings: 4

Ingredients

- 1 ½ cups beef stock
- 2 lb. of pork belly
- 4 tbsp. olive oil
- 1 batch low-carb Barbecue Dry Rub
- 2 tbsp. Instant Espresso powder

Directions

1. Preheat the broiler to 350°F.
2. Warmth the hamburger stock in a little pan over medium warmth until hot yet not bubbling
3. In a little bowl, combine the grill dry rub and coffee powder until very much joined.
4. Spot the pork midsection, skin side up in a shallow dish, and sprinkle 2 tablespoons of the olive oil over the top, scouring it over the whole pork tummy.
5. Pour the hot stock around the pork midsection and spread the dish firmly with aluminum foil. Prepare for 45 minutes. Cut into 8 thick cuts.
6. Warm the staying olive oil in a skillet over medium-high warmth and singe each cut for 3 minutes on each side or until the ideal degree of freshness is come to.

Nutrition

- Calories: 464
- Carbs: 3.4 g.
- Fat: 68 g.
- Protein: 24 g.

70. Herbed Chicken Breasts

Preparation time: 10 minutes
Cooking time: 40 minutes
Servings: 8

Ingredients

- 4 chicken breasts, skinless and boneless
- 1 Italian pepper, deveined and thinly sliced
- 10 black olives, pitted
- 1 ½ cups vegetable broth
- 2 garlic cloves, pressed
- 2 tbsp. olive oil
- 1 tbsp. Old Sub Sailor
- Salt, to taste

Directions

1. Rub the chicken with the garlic and Old Sub Sailor; salt to taste. Heat the oil in a frying pan over moderately high heat.
2. Sear the chicken until it is browned on all sides, about 5 minutes.
3. Add in the pepper, olives, and vegetable broth and bring it to a boil. Reduce the heat simmer and continue to cook, partially covered, for 30–35 minutes.

Nutrition

- Calories: 306
- Carbs: 3.1 g.
- Fat: 17.8 g.
- Fiber: 0.2 g.
- Protein: 31.7 g.

71. Cheese and Prosciutto Chicken Roulade

Preparation time: 15 minutes
Cooking time: 35 minutes
Servings: 2

Ingredients

- ½ cup Ricotta cheese
- 4 slices of prosciutto
- 1 lb. chicken fillet
- 1 tbsp. fresh coriander, chopped
- Salt and ground black pepper, to taste pepper
- 1 tsp. cayenne pepper

Directions

1. Season the chicken fillet with salt and pepper. Spread the Ricotta cheese over the chicken fillet; sprinkle with the fresh coriander.
2. Roll up and cut into 4 pieces. Wrap each piece with one slice of prosciutto; secure with kitchen twine.
3. Place the wrapped chicken in a parchment-lined baking pan. Now, bake in the preheated oven at 385°F for about 30 minutes.

Nutrition

- Calories: 499
- Carbs: 5.7 g.
- Fat: 18.9 g.
- Fiber: 0.6 g.
- Protein: 41.6 g.

72. Festive Turkey Rouladen

Preparation time: 15 minutes
Cooking time: 30 minutes
Servings: 5

Ingredients

- 2 lb. turkey fillet, marinated and cut into 10 pieces
- 10 strips prosciutto
- ½ tsp. chili powder
- 1 tsp. marjoram
- 1 sprig rosemary, finely chopped
- 2 tbsp. dry white wine
- 1 tsp. garlic, finely minced
- 1 ½ tbsp. butter, room temperature
- 1 tbsp. Dijon mustard
- Sea salt and freshly ground black pepper, to your liking

Directions

1. Start by preheating your oven to 430°F.
2. Pat the turkey dry and cook in hot butter for about 3 minutes per side.
3. Add in the mustard, chili powder, marjoram, rosemary, wine, and garlic.
4. Continue to cook for 2 minutes more.
5. Wrap each turkey piece into one prosciutto strip and secure with toothpicks.
6. Roast in the preheated oven for about 30 minutes.

Nutrition

- Calories: 286
- Carbs: 6.9 g.
- Fat: 9.7 g.
- Fiber: 0.3 g.
- Protein: 39.9 g.

73. Herby Chicken Meatloaf

Preparation time: 20 minutes
Cooking time: 30 minutes
Servings: 6

Ingredients

- 2 ½ lb. ground chicken
- 3 tbsp. flaxseed meal
- 2 large eggs
- 2 tbsp. olive oil
- 1 lemon, 1 tbsp. juiced
- ¼ cup chopped parsley
- ¼ cup chopped oregano
- 4 garlic cloves, minced
- Lemon slices to garnish, as desired

Directions

1. Preheat oven to 400°F. In a bowl, combine ground chicken and flaxseed meal; set aside. In a small bowl, whisk the eggs with olive oil, lemon juice, parsley, oregano, and garlic.
2. Pour the mixture onto the chicken mixture and mix well. Spoon into a greased loaf pan and press to fit. Bake for 40 minutes.
3. Remove the pan, drain the liquid, and let cool a bit. Slice, garnish with lemon slices, and serve.

Nutrition

- Calories: 362
- Fat: 24 g.
- Net carbs: 1.3 g.
- Protein: 35 g.

74. Garlic-Parmesan Chicken Wings

Preparation time: 10 minutes
Cooking time: 3 hours
Servings: 2

Ingredients

- 8 tbsp. (1 stick) butter
- 2 garlic cloves, minced

- 1 tbsp. dried Italian seasoning
- ¼ cup grated Parmesan cheese, plus ½ cup
- Pink Himalayan salt
- Freshly ground black pepper
- 1 lb. chicken wings

Directions

1. With the crock insert in place, preheat the slow cooker to high. Line a baking sheet with aluminum foil or a silicone baking mat.
2. Put the butter, garlic, Italian seasoning, and ¼ cup of Parmesan cheese in the slow cooker, and season with pink Himalayan salt and pepper. Allow the butter to melt, and stir the ingredients until well mixed.
3. Add the chicken wings and stir until coated with the butter mixture.
4. Cover the slow cooker and cook for 2 hours and 45 minutes.
5. Preheat the broiler.
6. Transfer the wings to the prepared baking sheet, sprinkle the remaining ½ cup of Parmesan cheese over the wings, and cook under the broiler until crispy, about 5 minutes.
7. Serve hot.

Nutrition

- Calories: 738
- Total fat: 66 g.
- Carbs: 4 g.
- Net carbs: 4 g.
- Fiber: 0 g.
- Protein: 39 g.

75. Braised Chicken Thighs With Kalamata Olives

Preparation time: 10 minutes
Cooking time: 40 minutes
Servings: 2

Ingredients

- 4 chicken thighs, skin on
- Pink Himalayan salt
- Freshly ground black pepper
- 2 tbsp. ghee
- ½ cup chicken broth
- 1 lemon, ½ sliced, and ½ juiced
- ½ cup pitted Kalamata olives
- 2 tbsp. butter

Directions

1. Preheat the oven to 375°F.
2. Pat the chicken thighs dry with paper towels, and season with pink Himalayan salt and pepper.
3. In a medium oven-safe skillet or high-sided baking dish over medium-high heat, melt the ghee. When the ghee has melted and is hot, add the chicken thighs, skin-side down, and leave them for about 8 minutes, or until the skin is brown and crispy.
4. Flip the chicken and cook for 2 minutes on the second side. Around the chicken thighs, pour in the chicken broth, and add the lemon slices, lemon juice, and olives.
5. Bake in the oven for about 30 minutes, until the chicken is cooked through.
6. Add the butter to the broth mixture.
7. Divide the chicken and olives between two plates and serve.

Nutrition

- Calories: 567
- Carbs: 4 g.
- Fiber: 2 g.
- Net carbs: 2 g.
- Protein: 33 g.
- Total fat: 47 g.

Fish Recipes

76. Salmon With Lime Butter Sauce

Preparation time: 20 minutes
Cooking time: 10 minutes;
Servings: 2

Ingredients

- 2 salmon fillets
- 1 lime, juiced, divided
- ½ tbsp. minced garlic
- 3 tbsp. butter, unsalted
- 1 tbsp. avocado oil
- Seasoning:
- ¼ tsp. salt
- ¼ tsp. ground black pepper

Directions

1. Prepare the fillets and for this, season fillets with salt and black pepper, place them on a shallow dish, drizzle with half of the lime juice, and then marinate for 15 minutes.
2. Meanwhile, prepare the lime butter sauce and for this, take a small saucepan, place it over medium-low heat, add butter, garlic, and half of the lime juice, stir until mixed, and then bring it to a low boil, set aside until required.
3. Then take a medium skillet pan, place it over medium-high heat, add oil and when hot, place marinated salmon in it, cook for 3 minutes per side and then transfer to a plate.
4. Top each salmon with prepared lime butter sauce and then serve.

Nutrition

- Calories: 192
- Fat: 18 g.
- Fiber: 0 g.
- Net carb: 4 g.
- Protein: 6 g. Salmon With Roasted Veggies

Preparation time: 10 minutes
Cooking time: 15 minutes;
Servings: 2

Ingredients

- 2 fillets of salmon
- 4 oz. asparagus spears cut
- 2 oz. sliced mushrooms
- 2 oz. grape tomatoes
- 2 oz. basil pesto

For the seasoning:

- ⅔ tsp. salt
- ½ tsp. ground black pepper
- 1 tbsp. mayonnaise
- 2 oz. grated mozzarella cheese
- 2 tbsp. avocado oil

Directions

1. Turn on the oven, then set it to 425°F and let it preheat.
2. Take a medium baking sheet lined with parchment paper, place salmon fillets on it and then season with ⅓ tsp. salt and ¼ tsp. ground black pepper.
3. Take a small bowl, mix together mayonnaise and pesto in it until combined, spread this mixture over seasoned salmon, and then top evenly with cheese.
4. Take a medium bowl, place all the vegetables in it, season with remaining salt and black pepper, drizzle with oil, and toss until coated.
5. Spread vegetables around prepared fillets and then bake for 12–15 minutes until fillets have thoroughly cooked.
6. Serve.

Nutrition

- Calories: 571
- Fat: 45.4 g.
- Protein: 34.1 g.
- Net carb: 3.5 g.
- Fiber: 2.2 g.

77. **Cheesy Baked Mahi-Mahi**

Preparation time: 10 minutes
Cooking time: 25 minutes;
Servings: 2

Ingredients

- 2 fillets of mahi-mahi
- ½ tsp. minced garlic

- 2 tbsp. mayonnaise
- 1 tbsp. grated Parmesan cheese
- 1 tbsp. grated mozzarella cheese

For the seasoning:

- ½ tsp. salt
- ¼ tsp. ground black pepper
- 1 tbsp. mustard paste
- ¼ of lime, juiced

Directions

1. Turn on the oven, then set it to 400°F and let it preheat.
2. Meanwhile, take a baking sheet, line it with foil, place fillets on it and then season with salt and black pepper.
3. Take a small bowl, add mayonnaise, stir in garlic, lime juice, and mustard until well mixed, and then spread this mixture evenly on fillets.
4. Stir Parmesan cheese and mozzarella cheese, sprinkle it over the fillets, and then bake for 15–20 minutes until thoroughly cooked.
5. Then turn on the broiler and continue cooking the fillets for 2–3 minutes until the top is nicely golden brown.
6. Serve.

Nutrition

- Calories: 241
- Fat: 13.6 g.
- Fiber: 0 g.
- Net carb: 1.1 g.
- Protein: 25 g.

78. Zucchini Noodles in Creamy Salmon Sauce

Preparation time: 5 minutes;
Cooking time: 7 minutes;
Servings: 2

Ingredients

- 3 oz. smoked salmon
- 1 zucchini, spiralized into noodles
- 1 tbsp. chopped basil
- 2 oz. whipping cream
- 2 oz. cream cheese, softened
- Seasoning:
- ⅓ tsp. salt
- ⅓ tsp. ground black pepper
- 1 tbsp. avocado oil

Directions

1. Cut zucchini into noodles, place them into a colander, sprinkle with some salt, toss until well coated, and set aside for 10 minutes.
2. Meanwhile, take a small saucepan, place it over medium-low heat, add whipped cream in it, add cream cheese, stir until mixed, bring it to a simmer, and cook for 2 minutes or more until smooth.
3. Then switch heat to low heat, add basil into the pan, cut salmon into thin slices, add to the pan, season with ¼ tsp. of each salt and black pepper and cook for 1 minute until hot, set aside until required.
4. Take a medium skillet pan, place it over medium-high heat, add oil and when hot, add zucchini noodles and cook for 1–2 minutes until fried.
5. Season zucchini with the remaining salt and black pepper and then distribute zucchini between two plates.
6. Top zucchini noodles with salmon sauce and then serve.

Nutrition

- Calories: 271
- Fat: 22 g.
- Fiber: 1.5 g.
- Net carb: 4.5 g.
- Protein: 13.5 g.

79. Sushi Shrimp Rolls

Preparation time: 2 minutes
Cooking time: 10 minutes
Servings: 5

Ingredients

- 2 cups cooked and chopped shrimp
- 1 tbsp. sriracha sauce
- ¼ cucumber, julienned
- 5 hand roll nori sheets
- ¼ cup mayonnaise

Directions

1. Combine shrimp, mayonnaise, cucumber, and sriracha sauce in a bowl. Layout a single nori sheet on a flat surface and spread about 1/5 of the shrimp mixture.
2. Roll the nori sheet as desired. Repeat with the other ingredients.
3. Serve with sugar-free soy sauce.

Nutrition

- Calories: 216
- Fat: 10 g.
- Net carbs: 1 g.
- Protein: 18.7 g.

80. Grilled Shrimp With Chimichurri Sauce

Preparation time: 10 minutes
Cooking time: 45 minutes
Servings: 4

Ingredients

- 1 lb. shrimp, peeled and deveined
- 2 tbsp. olive oil
- Juice of 1 lime
- Chimichurri
- ½ tsp. salt
- ¼ cup olive oil
- 2 garlic cloves
- ¼ cup red onions, chopped
- ¼ cup red wine vinegar
- ½ tsp. pepper
- 2 cups parsley
- ¼ tsp. red pepper flakes

Directions

1. Process the chimichurri ingredients in a blender until smooth; set aside. Combine shrimp, olive oil, and lime juice, in a bowl, and let marinate in the fridge for 30 minutes.
2. Preheat your grill to medium. Add shrimp and cook for about 2 minutes per side.
3. Serve shrimp drizzled with the chimichurri sauce.

Nutrition

- Calories: 283
- Fat: 20.3 g.
- Net carbs: 3.5 g.
- Protein: 16 g

81. Coconut Crab Patties

Preparation time: 3 minutes
Cooking time: 15 minutes
Servings: 8

Ingredients

- 2 tbsp. coconut oil
- 1 tbsp. lemon juice
- 1 cup lump crab meat
- 2 tsp. Dijon mustard
- 1 egg, beaten
- 1 ½ tbsp. coconut flour

Directions

1. In a bowl to the crabmeat, add all the ingredients, except for the oil; mix well to combine. Make patties out of the mixture.
2. Melt the coconut oil in a skillet over medium heat.
3. Add the crab patties and cook for about 2–3 minutes per side.

Nutrition

- Calories: 215
- Fat: 11.5 g.
- Net carbs: 3.6 g.
- Protein: 15.3 g.

82. Shrimp in Curry Sauce

Preparation time: 3 minutes
Cooking time: 15 minutes

Servings: 2

Ingredients

- ½ oz. grated Parmesan cheese
- 1 egg, beaten
- ¼ tsp. curry powder
- 2 tsp. almond flour
- 12 shrimp, shelled
- 3 tbsp. coconut oil

For the sauce:

- 2 tbsp. curry leaves
- 2 tbsp. butter
- ½ onion, diced
- ½ cup heavy cream
- ½ oz. cheddar cheese, shredded

Directions

1. Combine all dry ingredients for the batter. Melt the coconut oil in a skillet over medium heat. Dip the shrimp in the egg first, and then coat with the dry mixture. Fry until golden and crispy.
2. In another skillet, melt butter. Add onion and cook for 3 minutes. Add curry leaves and cook for 30 seconds. Stir in heavy cream and cheddar and cook until thickened.
3. Add shrimp and coat well. Serve.

Nutrition

- Calories: 560
- Fat: 41 g.
- Net carbs: 4.3 g.
- Protein: 24.4 g.

83. Tilapia With Olives and Tomato Sauce

Preparation time: 5 minutes
Cooking time: 25 minutes
Servings: 4

Ingredients

- 4 tilapia fillets
- 2 garlic cloves, minced
- 2 tsp. oregano
- 14 oz. diced tomatoes
- 1 tbsp. olive oil
- ½ red onion, chopped
- 2 tbsp. parsley
- ¼ cup Kalamata olives

Directions

1. Heat olive oil in a skillet over medium heat and cook the onion for 3 minutes.
2. Add garlic and oregano and cook for 30 seconds.
3. Stir in tomatoes and bring the mixture to a boil. Reduce the heat and simmer for 5 minutes.
4. Add olives and tilapia, and cook for about 8 minutes. Serve the tilapia with tomato sauce.

Nutrition

- Calories: 282
- Fat: 15 g.
- Net carbs: 6 g.
- Protein: 23 g.

84. Lemon Garlic Shrimp

Preparation time: 2 minutes
Cooking time: 20 minutes
Servings: 6

Ingredients

- ½ cup butter, divided
- 2 lb. shrimp, peeled and deveined
- Salt and black pepper to taste
- ¼ tsp. sweet paprika
- 1 tbsp. minced garlic
- 3 tbsp. water
- 1 lemon, zested and juiced
- 2 tbsp. chopped parsley

Directions

1. Melt half of the butter in a large skillet over medium heat, season the shrimp with salt, black pepper, paprika, and add to the butter. Stir in the garlic and cook the shrimp for 4 minutes on both sides until pink. Remove to a bowl and set aside.

2. Put the remaining butter in the skillet; include the lemon zest, juice, and water. Add the shrimp, parsley, and adjust the taste with salt and pepper. Cook for 2 minutes. Serve shrimp and sauce with squash pasta.

Nutrition

- Calories: 258
- Fat: 22 g.
- Net carbs: 2 g.
- Protein: 13 g.

85. Baked Haddock

Preparation time: 10 minutes
Cooking time: 30 minutes
Servings: 2

Ingredients

- ½ lb. haddock
- 1 ½ tsp. water
- 1 tbsp. lemon juice
- Salt and black pepper to taste
- 1 tbsp. mayonnaise
- ½ tsp. dill weed
- Cooking spray
- Pinch of old bay seasoning

Directions

1. Spray a baking dish with cooking oil.
2. Add lemon juice, water, and fish and toss to coat.
3. Add salt, pepper, old bay seasoning, and dill weed, and toss again.
4. Add mayo and spread well.
5. Bake in the oven at 350°F for 30 minutes.
6. Serve.

Nutrition

- Calories: 104
- Carb: 0.5 g.
- Fat: 12 g.
- Protein: 20 g.

86. Trout With Sauce

Preparation time: 1 minute
Cooking time: 10 minutes
Servings: 2

Ingredients

- 2 big trout fillets
- Salt and black pepper to taste
- 2 tbsp. olive oil
- 2 tbsp. ghee
- Zest and juice from 2 oranges
- 2 handful parsley, chopped
- 1 cup pecans, chopped

Directions

1. Heat a pan with oil over medium-high heat.
2. Add the fish fillet and season with salt and pepper.
3. Cook for 4 minutes on each side. Transfer to a plate and keep warm.
4. Heat the same pan with the ghee over medium heat, then add the pecans. Stir and toast for 1 minute.
5. Add orange juice and zest, some salt and pepper, and chopped parsley.
6. Stir and cook for 1 minute.
7. Pour the mixture over the fish fillet. Serve.

Nutrition

- Calories: 200
- Carb: 1 g.
- Fat: 10 g.
- Protein: 14 g.

87. Roasted Salmon With Kimchi

Preparation time: 10 minutes
Cooking time: 2-10 minutes
Servings: 2

Ingredients

- 1 tbsp. ghee, soft
- ½ lb. salmon fillets
- 1 oz. kimchi, finely chopped

- Salt and black pepper to taste

Directions

1. In the food processor, mix ghee with kimchi and blend well.
2. Rub salmon with salt, pepper, and kimchi mix and place into a baking dish.
3. Place in the oven and bake at 425°F for 15 minutes.
4. Serve.

Nutrition

- Calories: 200
- Fat: 12 g.
- Carb: 3 g.
- Protein: 21 g.

88. Parmesan Crusted Salmon

Preparation time: 10 minutes
Cooking time: 15 minutes
Servings: 2

Ingredients

- 1 ½ garlic cloves, minced
- 1 lb. salmon fillet
- Salt and black pepper to taste
- ¼ cup parmesan, grated
- ⅛ cup parsley, chopped

Directions

1. Place the salmon on a lined baking sheet. Season with salt, and pepper. Cover with parchment paper.
2. Place in the oven at 425°F and bake for 10 minutes.
3. Remove the fish and sprinkle with Parmesan, parsley, and garlic.
4. Bake again for 5 minutes.
5. Serve.

Nutrition

- Calories: 240
- Fat: 12 g.
- Carb: 0.6 g.
- Protein: 25 g.

Superfoods for Women Over 50

89. Almond Brittles

Preparation time: 10 minutes
Cooking time: 15 minutes
Servings: 4

Ingredients

- 2 cup almonds
- ¼ cup butter
- ½ cup Swerve
- 2 tsp. organic vanilla extract
- ¼ tsp. salt
- ⅛ tsp. coarse salt

Directions

1. Line a 9x9-inch cake pan using parchment paper.
2. Add the butter, Swerve, vanilla, and ¼ teaspoon of salt in an 8-inch nonstick skillet over medium heat and cook until well combined, stirring continuously.
3. Stir in the almonds and bring to a boil, stirring continuously.
4. Cook for about 2–3 minutes, stirring continuously.
5. Remove the skillet from heat and place the mixture evenly into the prepared pan.
6. With the back of a spoon, stir to spread the almonds and sprinkle with salt.
7. Set aside for about 1 hour or until cooled completely.
8. Break into pieces and serve.

Nutrition

- Calories: 130
- Protein: 1.79 g.
- Fat: 13.18 g.
- Carbohydrates: 0.34 g.

90. Bacon Pickle Fries

Preparation time: 10 minutes
Cooking time: 15 minutes
Servings: 12

Ingredients

- 12 slices bacon
- 12 pickle spears
- ¼ cup intermittent-friendly-ranch dressing

Directions

1. Set the oven at 425°F.
2. Prepare a baking tin using a layer of parchment baking paper.
3. Wrap each of the pickles using a piece of bacon and arrange them on the prepared baking tray.
4. Bake until crispy (12–15 min.). Turn after about halfway through the cycle (7 min.).
5. Serve with your favorite ranch or other dressing.

Nutrition

- Calories: 159
- Net carbohydrates: 1.2 g.
- Protein: 2 g.
- Total fat: 16 g.

91. Broiled Bacon Wraps With Dates

Preparation time: 10 minutes
Cooking time: 15–20 minutes
Servings: 6

Ingredients

- 1 lb. sliced bacon
- 8 oz. pitted dates

Directions

1. Warm up the oven to reach 425°F.
2. Use a ½ slice of bacon and wrap each of the dates. Close with a toothpick.
3. Put the wraps on a baking tray and bake them for 15–20 minutes. Serve hot.

Nutrition

- Calories: 203
- Net carbohydrates: 5 g.
- Protein: 19 g.
- Total fat: 10 g.

92. Salmon Mascarpone Balls

Preparation time: 7 minutes
Cooking time: 0 minutes
Servings: 6

Ingredients

- 3 oz. smoked salmon, chopped
- 3 oz. mascarpone
- ½ tsp. maple flavor
- ½ tsp. chives, chopped
- 3 tbsp. hemp hearts

Directions

1. In a small food processor, combine salmon, mascarpone, maple flavor, and chives. Pulse a few times until blended together.
2. Form mixture into 6 balls.
3. Put hemp hearts on a medium plate and roll individual balls through to coat evenly.
4. Serve immediately or refrigerate for up to 3 days.

Nutrition

- Calories: 65
- Fat: 5 g.
- Net carbs: 0 g.
- Protein: 3 g.
- Total carbs: 1 g.

93. Bacon, Artichoke, and Onion Fat Bombs

Preparation time: 15 minutes
Cooking time: 8 minutes
Servings: 4

Ingredients

- 2 bacon slices
- 2 tbsp. ghee
- ½ large onion, peeled, diced
- 1 garlic clove, minced
- ⅓ cup canned artichoke hearts, sliced
- ¼ cup sour cream
- ¼ cup mayonnaise

- 1 tbsp. lemon juice
- ¼ cup Swiss cheese, grated
- Salt, pepper to taste
- 4 avocado halves, pitted

Directions

1. In a hot skillet, fry the bacon for 5 minutes. Let cool, then crumble.
2. Cook the onion and garlic using ghee for 3 minutes.
3. Combine the onion and garlic with the bacon and the remaining ingredients. Mix well. Season with salt and pepper. Refrigerate for 30 minutes. Fill the avocado halves with the mixture and serve.

Nutrition

- Calories: 408
- Fat: 39.6 g.
- Net carbs: 4 g.
- Protein: 6.6 g.
- Total carbs: 10 g.

94. Chocolate Shakes

Preparation time: 10 minutes
Cooking time: 0 minutes
Servings: 2

Ingredients

- 4 oz. coconut milk
- ¾ cup heavy whipping cream
- 1 tbsp. Swerve natural sweetener
- ¼ tsp. vanilla extract
- 2 tbsp. unsweetened cocoa powder

Directions

1. Empty the cream into a cold metal bowl. Use your hand mixer and chilled beaters to form stiff peaks.
2. Slowly add the milk into the cream. Add in the rest of the ingredients.
3. Stir well and pour into two frosty glasses. Chill in the freezer one hour before serving. Stir several times.

Nutrition

- Calories: 210
- Net carbohydrates: 7 g.
- Protein: 4 g.
- Total fat: 47 g.

95. Strawberry Almond Smoothie

Preparation time: 10 minutes
Cooking time: 0 minutes
Servings: 2

Ingredients

- ¼ cup frozen unsweetened strawberries
- 2 tbsp. whey vanilla isolate powder
- ½ cup heavy cream
- 16 oz. unsweetened almond milk
- Stevia (as desired)

Directions

1. Toss or pour each of the ingredients into a blender.
2. Puree until smooth.
3. Pour a small amount of water to thin the smoothie as needed.

Nutrition

- Calories: 34
- Net carbohydrates: 7 grams
- Protein: 15 g.
- Total fat: 25 g.

96. Salted Caramel and Brie Balls

Preparation time: 5 minutes
Cooking time: 5 minutes
Servings: 6

Ingredients

- 4 oz. brie, roughly chopped
- 2 oz. salted macadamia nuts
- ½ tsp. caramel flavor
- 1 tbsp. butter
- 1 large apple, chopped

Directions

1. In a food processor, mix all ingredients until a coarse mix forms, about 30 seconds.
2. Form mixture into 6 balls.
3. In a saucepan, melt the butter, then add the chopped apples.
4. Cook the apples for about 5 minutes.
5. Spoon the apples over the brie balls. Serve or refrigerate for up to 3 days.

Nutrition

- Calories: 130
- Fat: 12 g.
- Net carbs: 0 g.
- Protein: 5 g.
- Total carbs: 1 g.

97. **Intermittent Popcorn Cheese Puffs**

Preparation time: 5 minutes
Cooking time: 5 minutes
Servings: 4

Ingredients

- 4 oz. cheddar cheese sliced

Directions

1. Cut the cheddar into little ¼-inch squares.
2. Cover the pan with baking parchment.
3. Leave the cheddar to dry out for in any event 24 hours.
4. The following day preheat your oven to 390°F and heat the cheddar for 3–5 minutes until it is puffed up.
5. Leave to cool for 10 minutes before serving.

Nutrition

- Calories: 114
- Carbs: 2.2 g.
- Fat: 9 g.
- Protein: 7 g.

98. **Parmesan Vegetable Crips**

Preparation time: 5 minutes
Cooking time: 10 minutes
Servings: 4

Ingredients

- ¾ cup shredded zucchini
- ¼ cup shredded carrots
- 2 cups shredded Parmesan cheese
- 1 tbsp. olive oil
- ¼ tsp. black pepper

Directions

1. Set the oven to 375°F. Arrange a cookie tray with parchment paper.
2. Wrap shredded vegetables in a paper towel and remove excess moisture.
3. Mix all ingredients in a bowl and mix well.
4. Put tbsp. sized mounds onto the prepared cookie sheet.
5. Bake for 7–10 minutes until lightly browned.
6. Let it cool for at least 2–3 minutes and serve.

Nutrition

- Calories: 206
- Carbs: 3.6 g.
- Fat: 14.1 g.
- Protein: 15.8 g.

99. **Nori Snack Rolls**

Preparation time: 5 minutes
Cooking time: 10 minutes
Servings: 4

Ingredients

- 2 tbsp. almond, cashew, peanut, or another nut butter
- 2 tbsp. tamari, or soy sauce
- 4 standard nori sheets

- 1 mushroom, sliced
- 1 tbsp. pickled ginger
- ½ cup grated carrots

Directions

1. Set the oven to 350°F. Combine together the nut butter and tamari until smooth and very thick. Layout a nori sheet, rough side up, the long way.
2. Spread a thin line of the tamari mixture on the far end of the nori sheet, from side to side.
3. Lay the mushroom slices, ginger, and carrots in a line at the other end (the end closest to you).
4. Fold the vegetables inside the nori, rolling toward the tahini mixture, which will seal the roll. Repeat to make 4 rolls.
5. Bring on a baking sheet, then bake for 8–10 minutes, or the rolls are slightly browned and crispy at the ends. Let the rolls cool for a few minutes, then slice each roll into 3 smaller pieces.

Nutrition

- Calories: 79
- Carbs: 6 g.
- Fiber: 2 g.
- Protein: 4 g.
- Total fat: 5 g.

100. Risotto Bites

Preparation time: 15 minutes
Cooking time: 20 minutes
Servings: 12

Ingredients

- ½ cup bread crumbs
- 1 tsp. paprika
- 1 tsp. chipotle powder or ground cayenne pepper
- 1 ½ cups cold Green Pea Risotto
- Nonstick cooking spray

Directions

1. Set the oven to 425°F.
2. Line a baking sheet using parchment paper.
3. On a large plate, put and combine the panko, paprika, and chipotle powder. Set aside.
4. Make the 2 tablespoons of the risotto into a ball.
5. Roll in the bread crumbs, then put on the prepared baking sheet. Repeat to make a total of 12 balls.
6. Spray the tops of the risotto bites with nonstick cooking spray then bake for at least 15–20 minutes until it starts to brown. Cool it before storing it in a large airtight container in a single layer.

Nutrition

- Calories: 100
- Carbohydrates: 17 g.
- Fat: 2 g.
- Fiber: 5 g.
- Protein: 6 g.
- Sodium: 165 mg.
- Sugar: 2 g.

Chapter 12. 14 Days Meal Plan

Week 1

WEEK 1	11 PM–7 AM	MEAL 1	MEAL 2	MEAL 3
Day 1 (Sunday)	Fasting	Savory intermittent pancake	Beef, pepper, and green beans stir-fry	Cheesy baked mahi-mahi
Day 2 (Monday)	Fasting	Bacon and zucchini egg breakfast	Salmon with roasted veggies	Garlic-parmesan chicken wings
Day 3 (Tuesday)	Fasting	Spinach and eggs mix	Pork fillets with mustard sauce	Sushi shrimp rolls
Day 4 (Wednesday)	Fasting	Shrimp omelet	Zucchini noodles in creamy salmon sauce	Teriyaki beef stir-fry
Day 5 (Thursday)	Fasting	Sausage styled rolled omelet	Cheese and prosciutto	Chinese bok choy and turkey soup

134

			chicken roulade	
Day 6 (Friday)	Fasting	Savory ham and cheese waffles	Grilled shrimp with chimichurri sauce	Pork medallions with aromatic herb butter
Day 7 (Saturday)	Fasting	Sausage-stuffed bell peppers	Beef with cabbage noodles	Sunflower seeds and arugula garden salad

Week 2

WEEK 2	11 PM–7 AM	MEAL 1	MEAL 2	MEAL 3
Day 1 (Sunday)	Fasting	Zucchini pancakes	Braised chicken thighs with kalamata olives	Salmon with lime butter sauce
Day 2 (Monday)	Fasting	Chia breakfast bowl	Lemon garlic shrimp	Parmesan roasted cabbage
Day 3 (Tuesday)	Fasting	Bacon and zucchini egg breakfast	Parmesan crusted salmon	Intermittent rosemary roast beef and white radishes
Day 4 (Wednesday)	Fasting	Intermittent tacos with guacamole and bacon	Chicken salad in cucumber cups	Garlic 'n sour cream zucchini bake
Day 5 (Thursday)	Fasting	Sausage-stuffed bell peppers	Herbed chicken breasts	Trout with sauce

Day 6 (Friday)	Fasting	Shrimp omelet	Tilapia with olives and tomato sauce	Broccoli salad
Day 7 (Saturday)	Fasting	Savory ham and cheese waffles	Pork cutlets in chili tangy sauce	Cheesy roasted vegetable spaghetti

Chapter 13. FAQs

Is Intermittent Fasting Difficult to Adhere To?

It could be difficult for some people. You may experience difficulties and challenges especially if you are still a beginner and your body still adjust and adapts to the new routine and pattern of food intake. Once your body adapts, you will find the eating pattern more manageable and easier to follow.

The main premise is being more aware of when and what you should eat. With such awareness, you will know exactly the boundaries and limitations you have to keep in mind. Also, it would be best to pair this approach with daily exercise and make healthy food choices, like fruits, beans, veggies, healthy fats, lean proteins, and lentils.

Avoiding too much sugar and sodium is a must, too. Once your body adapts to these new guidelines, adhering to IF will no longer be that challenging.

What Is the Recommended Number of Hours/Days for Fasting?

In most cases, followers of the IF approach set their fasting window to up to 16 hours daily. Most follow this routine as it is a bit easy to adapt and adhere to. You can do it just by skipping breakfast after you ate your last meal the other day. If you can, you may also practice the IF pattern, which requires you to go without food for 24 hours straight twice every week.

Do I Still Need to Count Calories?

The answer to this will depend on the goals you want to achieve while practicing IF. It is not necessary in some cases but if your goal is to lose weight, then you may want to monitor your calorie intake still.

Also, if you plan to cut out on snacks before sleeping or go without eating for a long period, then you will notice your calorie count declining naturally. Another thing to note is that taking in foods that are mostly plant-based will also naturally lower your calorie intake.

Should Women Do IF Differently?

In most cases, men and women tend to respond differently to the IF protocol. Most women also agree that they tend to achieve better results by widening their eating window a bit. For instance, when trying to follow the 16/8 IF plan, some women noticed that they get better results after they modified the approach – that is increasing the number of eating hours to 10 and reducing the fasting hours to 14.

A wise tip is to experiment and find out which one works for you. Observe the signals and cues sent by your body. Determine how it reacts to a specific IF pattern, too. Make sure to stick to an approach that seems to stimulate positive and favorable responses from your body.

Is It Safe for Pregnant or Breastfeeding Women to Fast?

Intermittent fasting is not highly recommended for pregnant women. It is mainly because your focus during pregnancy should be to supply your body with nutrients that can support your health and the growth and development of your baby. You need to eat highly nutritious foods that will help develop and build your baby's body and brain.

Also, take note that there are pregnant women who have a hard time having enough iron stores. If you do not eat the required foods every day, then it might lead to iron deficiency, which is important for your baby. Despite that, there is still no rule that bans pregnant women from practicing IF.

If you are one of those who have already practiced it and your health is at its best, then following IF is most likely safe for you. Just make sure that you only do it after receiving consent from your doctor. Also, it would be best to shorten the fasting period. If you are used to doing it for 24 hours or more, then avoid doing it while you are pregnant. You should fast for at most 14–16 hours only.

If you are breastfeeding, long fasting periods also need to be avoided. It is because of the constant need for your baby for nutritional milk. Fasting may have a huge impact on the quality and production of breast milk so you have to be extra careful. A wise piece of advice is to avoid fasting for more than 12–14 hours if you are breastfeeding to ensure that the production of milk will not be interrupted.

Make sure to observe yourself and the body, too. If you notice that your milk supply suddenly dries up and you suspect that it is because of IF, then stop fasting right away. Try to eat more regularly to find out if doing so resolves the issue. If you notice fasting greatly hampering your milk production, then maybe it is time to stop it for a while and just continue once you have already stopped breastfeeding.

Can I Still Work Out Even If I Am Doing IF?

Of course, you can. If your fasting period is 24 hours or more, then you may want to schedule your workouts during your non-fasting days to ensure that you have more energy to complete the sessions. You can also see other women working out even during their fasting periods, especially if their fasting takes less than 24 hours.

It is because they notice how effective exercising during a fast is in building lean muscle mass. In general, you should schedule your exercise based on how your body feels as well as the workout habits you are used to.

Conclusion

Is Intermittent Fasting for You?

Intermittent fasting is an optimal tool to lead a healthy life. By following the principles of intermittent fasting, you can surely reach your goal of healthy and disease-free life. However, you must not see intermittent fasting just as a way to shed your extra pounds. Because intermittent fasting is not just a dieting method, it is a way of life.

Your body is a gift, and you need to take care of it. Excessive weight and obesity is surely a health issue that must be dealt with properly. And one of the right ways is intermittent fasting. Everyone has their capacity. Everybody is different with different needs and perspectives. This is the reason why intermittent fasting may not work for all of you. Therefore, you all must evaluate your body needs and stamina before setting on the journey of intermittent fasting. The intermittent fasting method is suitable for some people, while for others, it is not the right answer. You need to find out which category you belong to.

The most important thing to keep in mind while starting intermittent fasting is that you don't need to overburden yourself as this is not a matter of a few days or a few weeks. You have to adopt that method, which you can continue in the long run with the same consistency. Intermittent fasting is a lifestyle. So you have to adopt this lifestyle and get used to it. No one changes their lifestyle now and then. Start following this method; if you don't feel good about it, you can leave any time. The body is yours; hence the choice is all yours. However, don't jump to the conclusion hastily. You need to wait for a few days for results to show up. You will surely see positive changes in your body and mental health. Our bodies are designed in a way that they can adapt to the changes pretty quickly. You just need to train your body and mind to continue the process. Once your body gets the hang of it, there is no turning around. But if the method is not working for you, you can surely look for other alternatives out there.

Another important thing to keep in mind is the way you follow intermittent fasting. This method is all about restricting your mealtime around a certain period. So you must eat healthy and nutritious food during the eating time. A lot of people don't like the idea and think that it is difficult to follow. The answer to this problem is that fasting is surely difficult at the start but not impossible. Indolent and unhealthy lifestyle is at peak these days. We all spend our time watching television or scrolling through our phones. Our active time is much shorter that leads to body issues like weight gain and sometimes serious health problems like cardiac problems or diabetes. These problems can be overcome with the intermittent fasting method, in which not only, you have to restrict your meals, but also do regular exercise. In conclusion, you are in charge of your body, so you must make the best decision regarding your body, mind, and health.

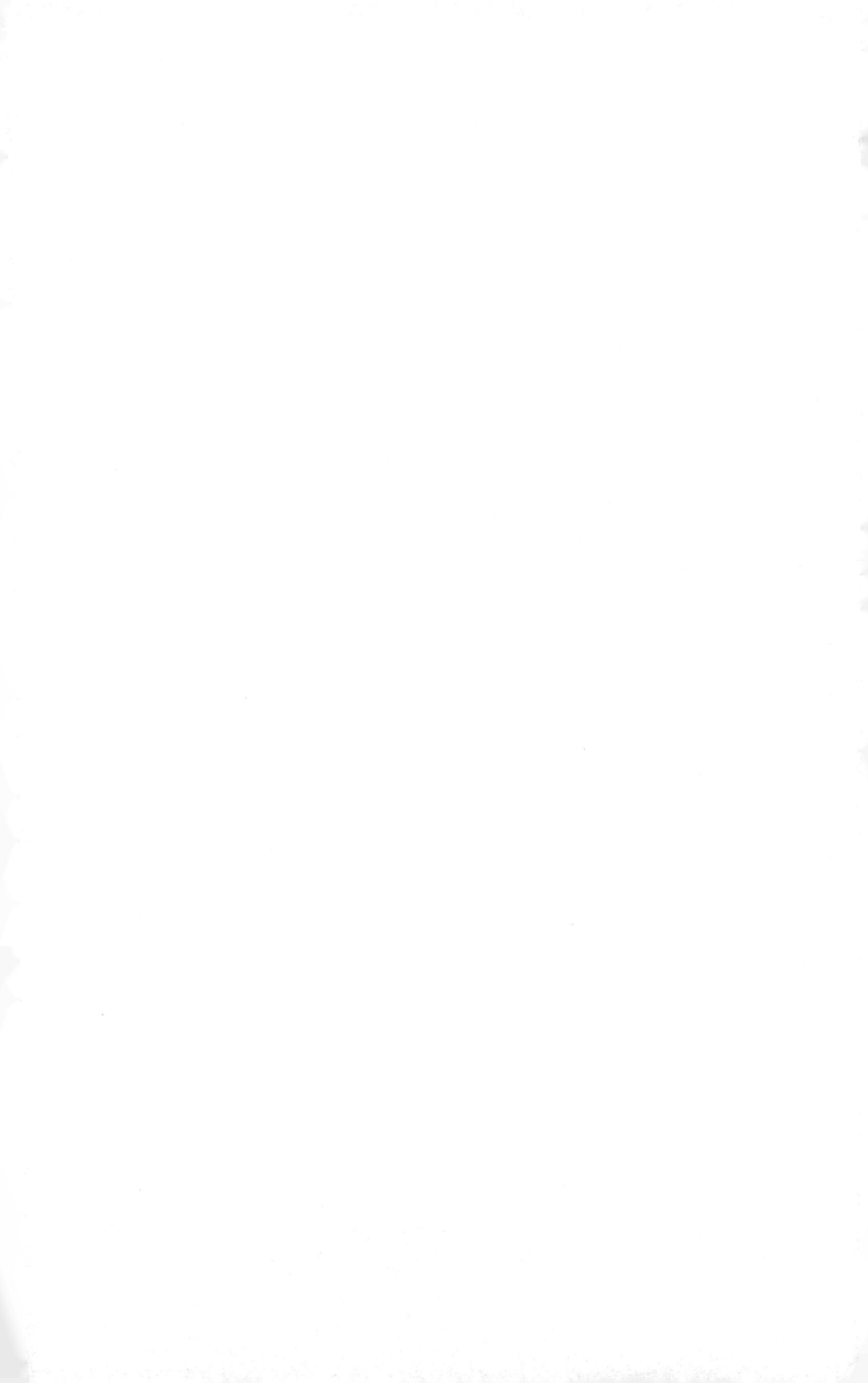

Printed in Great Britain
by Amazon